DR. MAROTTA'S ORGANIZED APPROACH

To OPTIMIZING

YOUR HEALTH

DR. MAROTTA'S ORGANIZED APPROACH to OPTIMIZING YOUR HEALTH

A HEALTH-CARE NAVIGATOR FOR THE LAYMAN

Joseph A. Marotta, M.D.

iUniverse, Inc.
New York Lincoln Shanghai

Dr. Marotta's Organized Approach to Optimizing Your Health
A Health-Care Navigator For the Layman

iUniverse books may be ordered through booksellers or by contacting:

iUniverse
2021 Pine Lake Road, Suite 100
Lincoln, NE 68512
www.iuniverse.com
1-800-Authors (1-800-288-4677)

Because of the dynamic nature of the Internet, any Web addresses or links contained in this book may have changed since publication and may no longer be valid.

The information, ideas, and suggestions in this book are not intended as a substitute for professional medical advice. Before following any suggestions contained in this book, consult your physician. Neither the author nor the publisher shall be liable or responsible for any loss or damage allegedly arising as a consequence of your use or application of any information or suggestions in this book.

ISBN: 978-0-595-41091-0 (pbk)
ISBN: 978-0-595-85450-9 (ebk)

Printed in the United States of America

CONTENTS

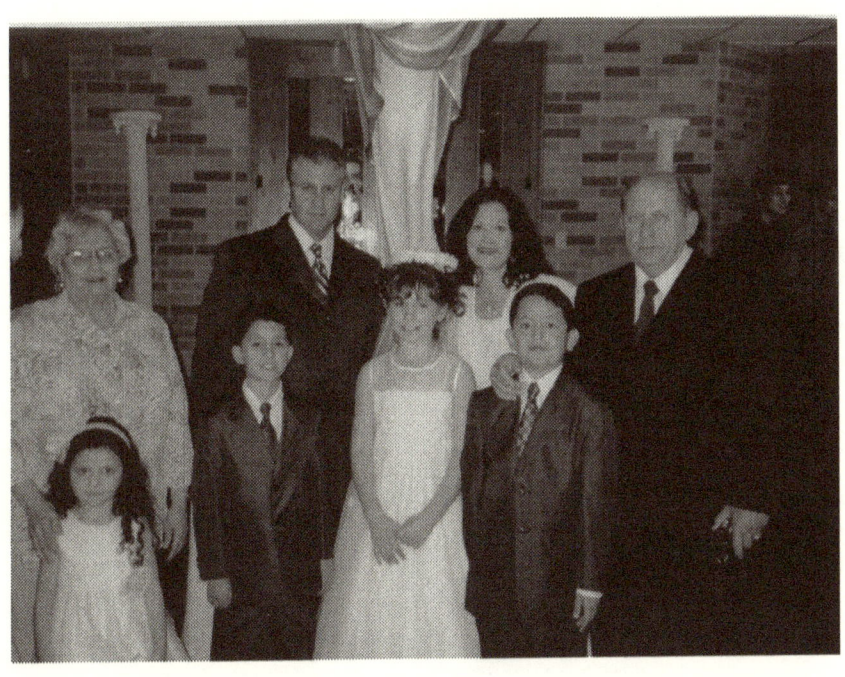

Meet "La Famiglia" (L-R) Back row, my mother Elsa,
yours truly, my wife Amanda, and my father Vincent.(L-R)
Front row, my children, Alessandra,
Thomas, Valerie, and Michael

PREFACE

If someone had told me when I was a fresh, young medical school graduate that I would someday write a how-to book on health optimization, I would have thought that they were crazy. For in July of 1995, as a brand new physician entering private practice, I was embarking upon yet another journey filled with the continuously evolving changes of the medical field. I had thought that after such a lengthy and intense education, there would be little in my future as a practicing physician that would compare with the rigors I had just survived. Not so! Although I can think of few endeavors that compare with the challenges of medical school and residency, a whole new aspect of medicine was awaiting my arrival. This was the nonacademic side of medicine; that is, the aspect of medicine that is not found in textbooks, lecture halls, or hospitals. I was to encounter this world head-on, as I had opted to enter private practice as a solo practitioner. I do not recall any courses in medical school which prepared me to know a good contract from a bad one or how to open up a private practice. I was not trained to do battle with insurance companies or HMOs that didn't care that I had not been reimbursed for services long-since rendered or of the high costs of malpractice insurance resulting from the enormous settlements awarded to the clients of blood-thirsty attorneys.

In spite of it all, I have managed to survive both the practice of medicine as well as the business end of medicine for over ten years now. For all of my success thus far I credit God, my parents, my personal family physician, and my wife who, to this very day, has never voiced a single complaint about my practice "taking up too much time." I also attribute a great deal of my motivation for practicing medicine to many of my attending physicians and upper-year residents at Temple University Hospital in Philadelphia, which residency I feel was the most rewarding aspect of my medical training. Other physicians with whom I have the privilege to associate in San Antonio continue to serve as role models for me to this very day.

One of the many observations that I have made in my clinical practice over the past ten years is that the biggest casualty of the increasing time constraints placed on the office visit is the doctor–patient relationship. This time constraint is the result of physicians' dependency on volume in order to compensate for decreasing reimbursement in an effort to survive in private practice. Due to these time constraints, and also in part due to the increasing complexity of medical technology, more and more patient questions go unanswered. In an effort to reduce the repercussions of limited time spent with the physician during doctor visits, I decided to write a small "patient guide" for my patients, filled with advice on frequently asked questions. These patient questions usually dealt with such matters as what to do in emergency situations and how to most quickly be seen by a physician when becoming acutely ill. Other aspects of this brief patient guide included tips on how to optimize the benefits of the doctor visit as well as how to select a health-care insurance plan and to optimize the benefits of pharmaceutical plans. At this point in time, the notion of writing a book designed to bridge the gap between patients and physicians crossed my mind, but because of a very busy inpatient and outpatient practice, I forced it temporarily to the back burner.

Shortly after writing my patient guide, I was approached by numerous pharmaceutical representatives to see if I had an interest in doing round table discussions with physicians regarding some of the latest treatments for various illnesses which were, for the most part, cardiovascular in nature. This seemed like an excellent opportunity to not only learn about pharmaceutical products but also to stay on the cutting edge of treatment. There was only one obstacle. For many years I had suffered from panic disorder or more specifically a social phobia when it came to public speaking. I was torn between my passion for medicine and my difficulty with public speaking. At this point, I decided to no longer be held a prisoner to fear of public speaking and meet it head on. To this day, I continue to deal with it and have tried to gain further insight into it by doing my own self-research.

One of the strong influences which helped me to go forth with doing presentations was the encouragement of a fellow physician/ nephrologist for whom I have the utmost respect who is a man by the name of Dr. Carl Dukes. Dr. Dukes' encouragement was particularly important to me as he himself was doing public speaking (mostly to physicians) except that he was on a national level. As a result of his encouragement and lots of prayer from my family and friends, I decided to proceed with it, social phobia or no social phobia. Needless to say, the round table discussions with fellow physicians have served to keep me on the cutting edge of medicine. One of the many concerns I had when beginning private practice was that I did not want to be a physician who does not keep up with the latest up-to-the-minute developments in medicine as it would make me a far less effective physician and by doing round table discussions/presentations with fellow physicians, this was far less likely to happen.

As a physician, I am responsible for keeping up with the latest advances in medical technology. As time went on, I realized that treating my own patients with these advances gave me great satisfaction. It is from this satisfaction that my dreams of writing this book finally came to fruition. This book was written in order to empower you, the reader, to take charge of your health. It is easy to read, filled with up-to-date information, and laid out in a simple step-by-step method covering a wide spectrum of topics that will help you navigate your way to optimal health through preventive medicine. The ultimate goals of optimal health are to live a longer and higher-quality life. In addition to providing a straightforward guide for taking charge of your health, I provide an age-group-specific checklist that will simplify and organize the process of optimizing your health. Throughout, an emphasis is placed on incorporating health-care-optimizing measures into today's world of medicine.

I recognize that the face of medicine has changed significantly, even in the past twenty years. When patients today refer to "my doctor" it is most commonly in reference to a group practice, or a staff of physicians. This very breakdown in patient-physician continuity (brought about by managed care for reduced costs and better care that have not been fulfilled) highlights again the need for individuals to take charge of their health-care outcomes. In today's world, physicians and patients alike continue to face the problem of time scarcity. The purpose of this book then, at least in part, is to serve as a supplement to the doctor–patient visit. The reality of today's world is that as a result of our advanced technology in the medical field, people are living longer. As a direct result of merely living longer, today's patients present us, their physicians, with multiple medication requirements, each of which address different medical problems. These medications are just a portion of what needs to be reviewed during the doctor–patient office visit. For the office visit, multiple factors need to be addressed, especially when the patient is visiting their primary care physician. The different portions of the doctor–patient visit include the following:

1. Describing the current complaint, that is, the reason that the patient presented for the office visit (which may be a follow-up or a new problem)

2. The maintenance portion which consists of reviewing the medications, noting which of them need new prescriptions, and then writing out those prescriptions

3. The health-maintenance portion which includes finding out what the patient's health-maintenance issues are and scheduling needed exams and tests

4. Filling out forms such as FMLA forms, signing for home health plans, signing for diabetic prescriptions, and completing other forms required for a variety of reasons.

The bottom line here is that because so many issues are expected to be addressed in such a brief period of time, it often becomes impossible to cover all of the bases. One solution is scheduling multiple appointments to address specific issues at different times.

Another important solution is one offered by this book, and that is to educate the patient about their health-maintenance issues. In an attempt to simplify the matter even further, I offer a checklist of the health-maintenance issues that need to be addressed by different age groups. For example, a 50-year-old female going to her annual checkup would most likely be in need of a Pap smear, mammogram, and colonoscopy. As a patient, these issues are made known to you by both reading the text portions of the book and by looking at the checklists provided.

In summation, at a time when doctor–patient visits are brief and very demanding, an easy-to-read, step-by-step guide that serves to optimize the practice of preventive medicine by educating patients is just what the doctor ordered. This book will hopefully lead to a significant reduction in morbidity (or occurrence of disease) and mortality (or occurrence of death) rates, allowing patients to live both higher-quality and longer lives.

CHAPTER ONE

OBJECTIVES OF BEING HEALTHY

The individual who coined the phrase, "If you have your health, you have just about everything" could not have spoken more truly. Unfortunately, more often than not, health is never appreciated enough until it begins to fail. Health is an ideal gauge when describing quality of life. I am sure that you can recall a particular rich, famous, or powerful person stricken by an incurable illness and the helplessness and pain which that particular illness inflicted. The illness cannot be remedied by any amount of money, influence, or power.

Being in good health is to an extent out of your control, but that is not what is important. What is important is that you recognize that the aspects of your health are twofold. There is a component of your health that is predetermined via heredity (whether in your favor or otherwise). In other words, you don't select your genetic makeup. However, it is your responsibility to deal with it. There is a second component of health, and unlike the first component, it is affected by your choices. This second component can best be described as lifestyle. There is no question that lifestyle can have a major impact on your health outcomes.

Guidelines which are associated with favorable cardiovascular health outcomes, for example, are first and foremost diet and exercise. In today's world of increasing incidences of hypertension, diabetes, dyslipidemia, and obesity, diet is of utmost importance. The increasing incidence of metabolic syndrome which is characterized by obesity with associated features such as diabetes, dyslipidemia, and high blood pressure in the United States is very alarming—particularly in children. The complications in a person's health brought on by diabetes can be devastating if the diabetes is uncontrolled, resulting in multiple organ involvement and its characteristic microvascular (small artery) and macrovascular (large artery) involvement. Hypertension is one of the most treatable risk factors for cardiovascular disease, but if uncontrolled, the risk of a cardiovascular event is incredibly high.

Hypertension also has a strong association with cardiovascular disease, particularly if uncontrolled. Therefore, in terms of dietary practices, it is necessary to control blood pressure via controlling sodium intake and controlling obesity. With regard to diabetes, carbohydrate intake and obesity are of utmost importance. Finally with regard to dyslipidemia, it is important to control intake of saturated fatty acids and cholesterol, as well as to control obesity.

Why is cardiovascular disease of such great importance?

The number one cause of death in the United States is cardiovascular disease. Approximately 1 million deaths per year are attributable to it. Approximately 2,600 people die every day in the United States as a result of cardiovascular disease. Cardiovascular disease is such a major cause of death that it by itself is responsible for more deaths per year than the remaining five other causes of death combined! Therefore, in order to make an impact on morbidity and mortality, it makes sense to target the most prevalent cause of death and any of the risk factors that are associated with it.

This being the case, what actions should be taken to optimize your health? The answer: pay a visit to a primary care physician, and have a thorough physical examination. A great deal of information may be obtained from this appointment. Important parameters which can be determined are blood pressure, diabetic state, cholesterol level, kidney function, liver function, and the presence of proteinuria (protein in the urine).

All of the above-mentioned diseases are risk factors for cardiovascular disease. Thus, if you are to optimize your health, control of blood pressure, diabetes, high cholesterol, and obesity would all be vital steps toward achieving this goal. Upon taking a closer look at hypertension, it is a known fact that uncontrolled hypertension is responsible in part for 370,000 deaths per year through its strong association with cardiovascular disease. On the other hand, if hypertension is controlled, clinical trials have shown statistically significant reductions in cardiovascular events, both fatal and nonfatal.

The tight control of blood pressure in diabetics has shown statistically significant reductions in both fatal and nonfatal heart attacks, strokes, heart failure, and limb amputations resulting from poor circulation. In addition, researchers have concluded through clinical trials that the administration of drugs called statins (cholesterol-lowering drugs) to patients who were not even hyperlipidemic but who had multiple risk factors resulted in a significant reduction in morbidity and mortality from cardiovascular disease. In one such study, which was terminated early due to such impressive results, the findings showed a 36% reduction in cardiovascular events and a 46% reduction in non-fatal myocardial infarction (heart attack) when hypertensive patients were treated with statins.

There are 45 million smokers in the United States today. The impact of smoking on morbidity and mortality is immense. Before going on any further, simply stated, smoking and tobacco use have yet to be associated with any favorable health outcome. Smoking is associated with cardiovascular disease, as well as cancer and lung disease. In terms of smoking's impact on morbidity and mortality, its strong association with cardiovascular disease, cancer, and pulmonary disease make it a very lethal risk. Simply put, if smoking doesn't give you a heart attack or stroke, it will give you lung cancer or emphysema. Chronic lower respiratory diseases are the third-leading causes of death in the United States.

Smoking doesn't only affect the individual who is doing the smoking, it also affects any close contacts, as many cases of smoking-related illnesses result from secondhand smoke inhalation. There have been countless numbers of cases of cardiovascular disease, lung cancers, and lung diseases associated with secondhand smoke inhalation.

In view of the big picture, the purpose of exercising preventive medicine is to live both a longer and higher quality of life. While some aspects of aging itself are not negotiable in terms of prevention and/or improvement, other aspects of aging can be improved upon with the final outcome being both a longer and a higher quality of life.

Preventive medicine hinges upon accomplishing the goals of a longer and higher quality of life. Primary care places a heavier emphasis on preventive medicine today than it has in years past. Medical technology has made tremendous strides in the last three decades, and it is on this cutting-edge technology and knowledge that the concepts of preventive medicine are based. The basis of preventive medicine is the identification of the risk factors of those conditions that cause death and the making of every effort to prevent them or at least slow their progression. By identifying and preventing those risk factors associated with the leading causes of death (which are cardiovascular disease, cancer, and stroke), we will make the greatest impact on morbidity and mortality, thus hopefully leading to both a longer and a higher quality of life.

Cardiovascular disease, as previously stated is by a large margin the leading cause of death in the United States. Cardiovascular disease by itself results in approximately 1 million deaths per year. This figure does not include cardiovascular events which do not result in death, such as non-fatal heart attacks or strokes.

Just what is cardiovascular disease? When I say cardiovascular disease, I am talking about myocardial infarction (or heart attacks), cerebrovascular accident (or stroke), congestive heart failure, and peripheral vascular disease. Peripheral vascular disease is the same process of narrowing of the arteries resulting from plaque build-up which results in heart attack and stroke. This pathological process, known as atherosclerosis or hardening of the arteries, occurs when cholesterol plaque accumulates within the inner lining (referred to as the "lumen"), narrowing the passage. This atheromatous plaque can become unstable, break off, and travel down an artery, eventually blocking the flow of blood and oxygen supply to a target organ. Hemoglobin, the oxygen transporter in the blood which carries the oxygen, becomes diminished as a result of diminished blood flow. The target organ which is being deprived of oxygen will begin to experience a deterioration in cell function, ultimately resulting in cell death if no other compensatory process takes place, such as help from neighboring vessels in what is known as "collateral circulation." This process of atherosclerosis can damage the heart, resulting in myocardial infarction, the brain, resulting in a stroke, or the extremities, resulting in gangrene and necessary amputations of partial or full extremities.

The impact of these cardiovascular events, even if they do not cause death, may still be devastating. This is the time when the quality-of-life issue surfaces. While amazing advances have improved the management of myocardial infarction, the aftermath can vary. The extent of the damage caused by the myocardial infarction may be minor, in which case, with medication, the patient may resume a close-to-pre-myocardial-infarction state. If the patient has suffered extensive myocardial damage, however, their quality of life may be altered by a significant reduction in cardiac function and consequently in levels of physical activity. Again, major advances have been made in the treatment of post-myocardial infarction, such as medications and placement of devices known as defibrillators. However, even a single experience of congestive heart failure reduces life expectancy.

The impact of a stroke (or a cerebrovascular accident) can be even more devastating than that of a myocardial infarction. The end results of a stroke may vary. It can be mild and the aftermath may be minimized with post-cerebrovascular-accident rehabilitation. On the other hand, the aftermath of a cerebrovascular accident may result in varying degrees of paralysis of a limb or limbs, diminished speech and swallowing function, as well as diminished (if not completely lost) cognitive function. An individual's loss of independence, which is all too often a byproduct of cerebrovascular accidents, is the ultimate illustration of quality of life reduction. This loss of quality of life carries with it not only the physical limitations brought on by the stroke, but also the mental, emotional, and financial repercussions which can be devastating.

The impact of peripheral vascular disease can be incredible. The pain of vascular compromise in an extremity can prove to be a tremendous burden on an individual. This can be relatively mild, such as the pain experienced in the calves while walking (known as intermittent claudication), which is treated with exercise and medication. It can also be severe, however, resulting in gangrene formation which can only be treated with amputation. The amputation, depending on the extent of the amputation and the amputation site, may result in the use of a limb prosthesis, requiring additional instructional physical therapy. This reduction in an individual's independence may result in severe mental, emotional, and financial hardships causing again a great deterioration in quality of life.

It is of the utmost importance to realize the immense impact of disease on the quality of life. For in today's world, length of life means little if it cannot be accompanied by quality of life. Therefore, our objectives are now more clear. We must take the necessary measures to both prolong life as well as to preserve the quality of life.

Just what are those measures which both prolong and preserve the quality of life? The initial step is to recognize that the leading causes of illness and death in the United States are cardiovascular disease, cancer, chronic lower respiratory disease, motor vehicle accidents, and diabetes mellitus. The next step would be to take the necessary precautions to minimize the risk of experiencing these disease states. Finally, we need to take the measures necessary to minimize the impact bought upon by the disease after it has occurred. (This is also known as secondary prevention.)

Upon reviewing the leading causes of death, it becomes evident why the focus of preventive medicine is on specific causes, particularly the more commonly occurring ones. Focusing on the most commonly occurring causes of death will yield the highest number of lives saved. Additionally, early detection is most likely to result in a more favorable outcome. Therefore, preventive medicine both attempts to prolong length of life as well as quality of life.

CHAPTER TWO

HOW TO CHOOSE YOUR DOCTOR

Choosing your physician may not be as important as choosing your spouse, but like choosing your spouse, it requires serious consideration. The criteria by which you choose your personal physician will certainly determine the quality of care that you receive. Situations often arise where important decisions concerning medical management need to be made. You must be confident that your physician will make decisions that are in accord with your wishes; medically sound; and carried out without undue influence of others.

Upon establishing a strong trust with a physician, scheduling an appointment to discuss your end-of-life decisions can prove to be a very productive session. Details regarding living wills can be established with clarity. By having such documents in writing with clarity, no obstacles stand in the way of decision making, nor should the appointed decision makers experience any confusion or guilty feelings. Having these legalities in order empowers the physician to make recommendations for his patients with greater clarity.

One of the most common reasons that patients become dissatisfied with their physicians is that they don't know what criteria to use when selecting their physician. To begin with, your primary care physician should be someone who listens to you, not just someone who hears you. Body language is important. Your physician must make good eye contact with you, as this conveys that he is listening and that what you are saying is important to him. It is also important that the physician sit down when talking to you, as this gesture suggests that he is not in a hurry and not trying to rush you. Other types of body language such as failing to sit down during a visit or repeatedly checking his watch, convey that your physician is hurried. However, you must realize that your physician does not have unlimited time. Be respectful of this.

Many patients prefer to speak to their physician personally when calling the office. Realistically, a busy physician often cannot return calls personally, as there is not ample time in a day. Calls returned by your physician should be restricted to those of major importance. If the calls can be fielded by office personnel, this is acceptable. If the request is too complicated or time consuming, scheduling an appointment is advised and if the situation is an emergency, the most appropriate action is to either call 911 or go to the emergency room.

Another common problem encountered by patients occurs when the patient becomes suddenly ill and wishes or needs to be evaluated by the physician. When selecting a physician, you must consider what options the physician offers when this situation arises. It is not acceptable to be told by the doctor's office that the next available appointment is in three to four weeks, as obviously by then you are either dead or have survived the current crisis. Ideally, a physician who tries his hardest to work you in within twenty-four to forty-eight hours is desirable. Again, in all fairness, the physician may be overloaded and simply unable to attend to all of his patients that day. This does not reflect poorly on the physician. However, look for office staffs that, upon instructions from the physician, provide reasonable options to you. For example, if the physician is unavailable, the office personnel may suggest that you go elsewhere that day where you can be attended to or offer to notify you in the event that another patient cancels an appointment that same day, so that you can be seen that same day.

There are situations where a patient becomes acutely ill and scheduling an appointment at the physician's office is not the best or most appropriate option. For example, if you develop acute onset chest pain and shortness of breath, the best advice would be to either call 911 or to have yourself transported to the nearest emergency room. Insisting on going to the physician's office, whether or not the physician is able to see you that day, may result in critical time lost which may greatly affect the outcome. Again, a physician's office that can provide sound advice is ideal.

Finally, there may be situations where you develop symptoms that may possibly be treated over the phone and medications called in to a pharmacy. This, of course, is at the discretion of a physician. This would obviously apply to an established patient, as it would be impossible to provide care to a patient unknown to a physician. If the physician feels comfortable enough to give medical advice over the phone or to call in prescriptions, it is most helpful to provide for the physician the most detailed description of your symptoms, such as fevers, chills, cough, shortness of breath, sore throat, and body aches, which greatly assists the physician in making a diagnosis and providing the most appropriate treatment.

So one of the criteria to consider when evaluating a physician is how responsive the physician and his office staff are to your needs. A physician who is unavailable is not a physician who is ideal for an individual. With all fairness, you cannot expect a physician to be available to personally assist you twenty-four hours a day and seven days a week, as this is not only unreasonable, but also impossible. However, a response to your needs which is both prompt and made with sound judgment is what is most important.

Another criterion which you need to consider when selecting a physician is continuity of care. This is obviously a personal decision. A physician may be part of a group or may be a solo practitioner. It is important to know if you will be seen by the same physician each time you schedule an appointment, as this may be of great importance to you and is oftentimes of little importance to HMOs and other insurance carriers. This is one of the many downsides of HMOs, as continuity of care, regardless of what they may say, is low on their priority list. Many patients find a level of comfort with a certain individual, and it becomes a major part of their healing process. It is ideal to select a physician who has an arrangement, whether part of a group or as an individual practitioner, which allows him or her to deliver this continuity of care. Obviously, you are most likely to encounter this continuity when being seen by a solo practitioner, although groups may have arrangements which prioritize continuity of care as well. The important thing is that you be informed of the arrangement prior to selecting a physician.

Another aspect of continuity of care regards hospitalization. You must become informed as to whether your physician follows patients who are hospitalized, as opposed to having another physician provide care in his place. Nowadays, doctors called hospitalists have emerged who provide this service for physicians who elect to devote their efforts to an outpatient practice exclusively. For some patients, having the primary care physician following them in the hospital is of great importance and something that should be considered greatly when selecting a physician. For others, continuity of care in the hospital setting may not be as important and therefore rank lower on their criteria list.

Feeling comfortable with a physician is oftentimes overlooked for numerous reasons but is nevertheless a very important criteria in selecting a physician. This level of comfort may be described as chemistry between the physician and patient. You as a patient need to have confidence in your physician and strongly believe that he or she will provide the best medical care for you. This is extremely important as it can reduce a great deal of the anxiety that can accompany a visit to the doctor's, both for you as well as your loved ones. Having this faith in your physician can be said to be part of the care itself which may quicken the recovery process.

It is of obvious importance in today's world of medicine to take into consideration whether or not your physician of choice accepts the health plan in which you are a participant. In reality, this should be the first on your list of criteria, as your medical expenses will be entirely out of pocket if the physician does not accept your health-care plan. If you do choose a physician that does not accept your plan, but cannot afford to pay for your medical expenses out-of-pocket, your options are to either select a physician who does participate in your health-care plan or to change health-care plans to one in which your preferred physician does participate as a provider. You must bear in mind that as most health-care plans work, if the primary care physician is not a participant, any referrals or ancillary tests such as CT scans, X-rays, and EKGs would also not be covered, as well as hospital admissions, which would leave you, the patient, with a very large bill. This is yet another undesirable aspect of managed care, but one that you must be aware of as part of the physician selection process in today's world.

There are services on the Internet which, for fees, provide information on physicians which may be important to you in deciding on a primary care physician. These fee-for-information services usually provide information on a physician's background, such as educational experience, board certification status, languages spoken, and the existence of any past litigation.

In summary, when selecting a primary care physician, some helpful hints which will enhance patient satisfaction are the following criteria:

- Have a strong belief that your physician will make medical decisions in your best interest and in accord with your wishes in the event that you become incapacitated, and who will work well with whomever is appointed with power-of-attorney.

- Feel comfortable with your physician. Find a physician who listens to your complaints and concerns with sincerity and who does not make you feel hurried. Be confident that your physician will act on those complaints and concerns.

- Receive prompt and satisfactory responses when becoming acutely ill while bearing in mind that this should be reserved for urgent situations. Other less-urgent situations or requests should be dealt with by scheduling a non-urgent appointment or not expecting an immediate response. Be aware that your physician is a human being and that he or she does not have unlimited time. Being considerate is always appreciated.

- Feel comfortable with the level of continuity of care provided by the physician. If you have a strong preference for continuity, select a physician whose style and availability provide that level of continuity in such ways as following patients both as inpatients and outpatients and in not having other physicians in his or her place on a constant basis.

- Find a physician in whom you can have strong faith and a physician with a favorable chemistry, as this criteria may strongly influence your recovery and strongly reduce anxiety for both you and your family and friends.

- Find a physician who participates in your health-care plan. This is mainly for financial reasons, which are also important to consider.

- Finally, if felt necessary, obtain via Internet services (for a fee) information on a physician's background which may assist you in making a primary care physician selection.

CHAPTER THREE

ACCESS TO HEALTH CARE

What exactly is meant by access to health care? A more understandable term could well be affordability of health care. How is this affordability obtained? There are numerous ways. There is always the plain and simple cash method, where services are obtained from a physician at a certain rate with the possibility of a discount for paying cash. The more common method is to have health insurance that, for a variable monthly premium, enrolls a patient in a plan that requires the patient to pay only a percentage of the cost of services or a co-pay, which is also variable. These services can be both inpatient and outpatient. Two methods of health-care finance are the Health Maintenance Organization (HMO) and the Preferred Provider Organization (PPO) plans. In an HMO/capitated plan, the physician may participate in a plan in which he is paid a flat rate per patient per month whether or not he provides services. A PPO is more similar to the conventional non-HMO health insurance plan. There may be other hybrid-like plans available as well. The most important aspects of acquiring access to health care are knowing how to distinguish a good plan from a bad plan and finding a plan that is affordable and most suited to you and your individual needs.

The simplest method of paying for health care is with good, old-fashioned cash. Some advantages to this method include the following:

- There are no monthly fees.

- There are no restrictions on access to providers—in other words, you can see the physician of your choice without being restricted to a limited panel by an insurance company or HMO.

- There are no formulary restrictions or necessary prior authorizations—in other words, as long as you are willing and able to pay the full price of a medication, there are no restrictions, provided you have a prescription from a physician.

- There are no restrictions on where a patient may seek outpatient or inpatient services—in other words, you can go to any hospital, laboratory, physical therapy, or radiology facility of your choice, provided that you are willing and able to pay for the services.

- Should you need referrals to another physician (presumably a specialist), there are no approvals processes that can cause delays or inconvenience to yourself.

In essence, in the event that a patient is capable of paying cash for services, all of the inconveniences brought upon by insurance companies and HMOs come to the surface. The opposites of all of the aforementioned conveniences of cash-paying patients are the inconveniences brought upon by insurance companies and HMOs for the sole purpose of increasing their revenues.

In today's world, however, the cash-paying patients make up a very small percentage of health-care users. The obvious reason being the cost of health care today. The cost of health care has skyrocketed over the years. There are multiple reasons for this skyrocketing increase. For starters, technology, while becoming increasingly sophisticated, has also become incredibly expensive. Hospitals charge astronomical fees as well for their services, and the cost of medications has also continued to rise. Ironically, in a world which views physicians oftentimes as the reasons for the high cost of health care, reimbursement to physicians has all but increased. In any event, the cash-paying patient, as a result of skyrocketing health-care costs, is clearly the exception rather than the rule.

So why do so many individuals obtain health insurance? This is simply a matter of logic—a situation of risks versus benefits. One has to weigh the risk of tragically needing hospitalization in which costs without insurance would be financially devastating against not needing or having little need for health care in which cash for services would be less expensive than the insurance premium. The risk of becoming incapacitated without a health-care plan will, more often than not, drive an individual to pay the high cost of an insurance premium. Becoming financially crippled as a result of a costly illness is too great a risk for most individuals to take.

So, as part of the vast majority of those who become enrolled in an insurance plan, where do you begin? First of all, you should be familiar with HMO and PPO which stand for Health Maintenance Organization and Preferred Provider Organization respectively. There are also other insurance programs which are neither HMO nor PPO but rather what would be referred to as hybrids. The HMO plans are usually the least expensive in terms of premiums although oftentimes the saying, "You get what you pay for" comes to mind when enrolling in an HMO program. HMO programs may be what are called capitated plans, in which a patient pays a certain monthly premium, and a physician is paid a flat amount per month whether she sees the patient zero times or thirty times. An HMO may also be a fee-for-service setup where a physician is paid a flat amount per patient visit whether complicated or simple—also for a fixed monthly premium. A PPO enrollment program is usually a fee-for-service setup. A PPO plan is usually more costly than an HMO. The advantages of a PPO over an HMO enrollment plan are usually several. PPOs usually allow the patient more autonomy, in that they usually have more participating Primary Care Physicians (PCP's) in the plan, allowing the enrollee a greater number of choices. PPO programs also may have no requirements for a referral to a specialist should their services be necessary. Not needing a referral usually will mean less paperwork and time lost, thus expediting services. Another advantage of the PPO over the HMO format in general is the prescription medication program. Although co-pays have continued to rise, PPO prescription plans usually provide at least partial coverage to a wider variety of medications.

It is highly advisable that you become as well-informed as possible regarding all forms of health-care plans. There are numerous health-care formats available and each plan offers a different spectrum of benefits. As mentioned earlier, it is in your best interest to be able to know the difference between a good plan and a bad plan. Most importantly, however, you must be able to determine and select a health-care program that is most appropriate for your own personal situation and needs. In selecting a health-care enrollment program, a checklist of benefits should be used as a guide so that you can make the most appropriate selection:

- Is the plan affordable? Unfortunately this is often the bottom line, because if a plan is not affordable, it matters little what it may offer. Unfortunately, costs for health-care plans only continue to rise, making it necessary for you to shop around for the best plan possible. One suggestion is to check for benefits offered by employers when seeking for employment, such as health insurance for both yourself and your family. You must bear in mind that getting insured through a group is usually less expensive, and pre-existing conditions may not be used against you as they otherwise may be when attempting to find a health-care plan as an individual. Although affordable health care is becoming more difficult to find, you must realize what the repercussions would be if you should need hospitalization, multiple medications, imaging studies, or inpatient or outpatient physical or occupational services. Without a health-care plan, the cost of such services could result in a financial disaster with longstanding repercussions. Therefore, some form of health-care plan is highly encouraged if at all possible for these reasons.

- Are there a reasonable number of physicians participating in the enrollment plan in the event that specialist services are needed? This is very important to consider as oftentimes the services of, for example, a cardiologist, nephrologist, or gastroenterologist, become necessary. The greater the number of participating specialists, the more choices you will have to select from, particularly if you have a preference. PPOs, in general, have a larger selection which likely contributes in part to the higher premiums (as compared to HMO plans which usually have a smaller selection of specialists).

- Does the health-care plan cover prescription medications? If so, what kind of coverage is offered? There are numerous prescription plan benefits, each with its unique spectrum of coverage. Some plans have deductibles, while others do not. Some plans have a tier-system co-pay which places generic brands, for example, on a tier-one level, trade-name medications (which are the more expensive "preferred" drugs) on a tier-two level, and the most expensive, only partially covered drugs on the tier-three level. In this system, the most expensive would be a medication which is not covered, for which the patient/enrollee would be paying 100 percent of the cost. It should also be mentioned that the prescription plans can be very deceiving, as the tier levels of a particular plan are subject to change at any time, which may work for you or against you. As a rule of thumb, the newer a medication is, the less likely it is to have good coverage, and the longer a medication has been around, the more likely it is to be either a tier three level or a tier two level, which provides better coverage.

Other types of prescription plan formats are those which offer a percentage-type coverage for a particular medication—for example, 25/75 or 30/70 or 50/50. If such is the case, it is highly recommended that you find the least expensive pharmacy, as this will minimize cost to yourself.

Finally, many insurance, HMO, and PPO plans are offering a three-month prescription format which is usually at a discounted rate. The way that this works is simple. If a patient/enrollee is on a medication taken regularly, say for example a medication for hypertension or high cholesterol, prescriptions are obtained from a physician allowing for receiving a three month supply of medication per prescription as opposed to the conventional one month supply per prescription. These are usually mailed out and received in the mail within two weeks. This format saves money in most cases, reduces trips to the pharmacy, and reduces pharmacy workload as well. Inquire about this benefit when deciding on a health-care plan, particularly if you are on medications that are taken regularly.

- Does the health-care plan provide coverage for services such as rehabilitation (inpatient and outpatient), skilled nursing facilities, home health care, and psychiatric services (inpatient and outpatient)? If so, you should also inquire about details such as deductibles, percent coverages/out-of-pocket expenses, and facilities that are within the network covered.

- Does the health-care plan provide partial coverage for out-of-network physician services and inpatient and outpatient facilities, and if so, what is the extent of coverage?

- What are the co-payment amounts for outpatient doctor visits; ancillary services, such as lab work; and radiological studies, such as X-rays, CT scans, MRIs, and sonograms?

- What is the inpatient cost format? Inquire about such aspects as the amounts of the deductible and/or percentage charges, if there are any.

- Does the plan have a reputation for requiring time-consuming, multi-step referral procedures which delay medical attention and shift the burden to the patient and the doctor?

- Does the plan provide coverage for durable medical equipment, such as wheelchairs, hospital beds, walking canes, and walkers? If so, are there any out-of-pocket costs, and if so, what are those costs?

- Does the plan provide coverage for needed health-maintenance procedures/studies such as colonoscopies? If so, how much coverage?

- Are there maternity services offered? If so, how much of the cost is covered?

- Are mammograms, PSA levels, and women's annual exams included, and if so, what is the extent of the coverage?

- Does the plan provide full or partial coverage for health-promoting measures, such as home gym equipment, health-club memberships, and weight reduction organization memberships?

- Does the plan cover bariatric surgeries, such as gastric bypass or lap band procedures for weight reduction, and if so, what are the criteria to qualify for the coverage?

- Does the health-care plan provide coverage for transportation, such as ambulance services when available?

All of the above are helpful hints that will assist you in obtaining a health-care plan that is most appropriate for meeting your specific needs.

CHAPTER FOUR

HOW TO GET THE MOST OUT OF YOUR DOCTOR VISIT

It has been said that "the wheel that never squeaks never gets greased." The same holds true when a patient presents for a doctor visit. Doctor visits are critical in determining how best to address your health issues and it is thus very important to get the most out of them. There are a number of helpful hints which you can apply that will optimize the benefits of a doctor visit.

It is always helpful to be prepared and organized. For example, if lab work is to be drawn, it is helpful to call the doctor's office in advance to see if you need to be fasting. This is important, because if certain laboratory studies are performed in a non-fasting state, the results will not be accurate. Examples of such results are fasting glucose levels and cholesterol panel studies. It is also important to know that certain laboratory studies do not require fasting. This is important, for example, because a diabetic may experience low blood sugars unnecessarily which may have negative outcomes, as they cannot tolerate long periods of time without eating.

When possible, it is helpful to have lab work done two to three days prior to your appointment, so that the results can be ready for review on the day of the appointment. This expedites your physician's ability to decide on your diagnosis and management, allowing results to be discussed immediately.

It is critically important that you either bring an accurate list of medications that you are on or that you bring the bottles of the medications themselves on the day of the doctor visit. This provides invaluable information to the doctor when deciding upon a treatment plan. This also reduces the workload and time consumed which can be better utilized in addressing your problems. In bringing the most recent prescription medication bottles, you can also determine which of the medications will require new prescriptions which can be addressed immediately as well. This reduces the office staff's workload, as they would not need to be calling the prescriptions in to the pharmacy.

In an effort to address as many problems as possible, it is advisable to write down a problem list so as to not forget to mention important problems. You must not get carried away with too many problems at once, however, as the physician's time is limited. In an effort to be fair, schedule another appointment to address the less-urgent problems, as once again, the physician is also a human being and if over-whelmed, may not be able to manage patients in an optimal manner. Consideration for the physician is both necessary and appreciated.

It is very helpful to have the name and telephone numbers of any other physicians that you have visited. This is particularly useful when presenting to a PCP (primary care physician) for the first time. In the event that reports of previous studies such as lab work, biopsies, mammograms, or operative reports are needed, they can more read-ily be obtained so as to avoid repeating costly studies unnecessarily as well as save time. Other helpful information would be reports of the results of previous studies such as echocardiograms, chest X-rays,

EKGs, and lab work which could be used as baseline studies to see if findings on new studies are new or already-addressed issues.

You can enable your physician to obtain your past medical history by signing a release which gives permission to another physician to release your medical records without violating privacy laws. Old records can greatly assist the doctor in providing the most appropriate care and in reducing the number of unnecessarily repeated studies, which in turn also reduces costs.

It is of utmost importance, particularly on the first office visit to provide the most accurate history regarding both your current and past medical problems. The bulk of information leading to a diagnosis is derived from an accurate history. Also, the more thorough and accurate the description of your ongoing problem, the fewer studies needed to come up with a diagnosis which, again, reduces costs and reduces delays in beginning treatment.

The more descriptive you can be during the office visit, the greater the likelihood will be of making the right diagnosis. There are simple hints that you may use when describing a medical problem. For example, when describing chest pain, it is important to describe the location of the pain; whether or not the pain is localized or radiates elsewhere, such as to the back, shoulder, arm, or jaw; associated symptoms, such as dizziness, diaphoresis (sweating), nausea, or palpitations; whether any measures taken, such as taking deep breaths, either improve or worsen symptoms; whether the current symptoms are new or old; and whether or not any previous treatments have been attempted and if those treatments have been successful. These helpful hints will optimize the likelihood of reaching a correct diagnosis which will result in minimal delay in providing the most appropriate treatment.

Also of utmost importance, particularly on the first visit, is an accurate and detailed history of your past health. You should be prepared to provide information regarding ongoing medical problems. For example, if you are diabetic, helpful information regarding the diabetes would include the following:

- When was it diagnosed?
- What medications, if any, are being taken to treat it?
- Is diet and exercise part of the current treatment plan?
- Are any recent laboratory study results such as a hemoglobin A_{1C} available?
- Has hospitalization been necessary in the past to manage the diabetes?

The answers to these questions will help guide the physician in deciding upon an optimal management plan.

When describing past surgical history, helpful information for the physician would include the following:

- The date of the surgery
- The hospital in which the surgery was performed
- The name(s) of the surgeon(s) who performed the procedure
- A detailed account of the surgery which could be obtained via an official operative report from the surgeon
- Whether or not any complications were encountered during this surgery

In reference to female patients, there are a number of important aspects of history which are relevant to the PCP. For instance, it is important to relay the number of times you have been pregnant. It is also important to provide to the physician the number of successful and unsuccessful pregnancies which may include miscarriages, total pregnancies, abortions, and still births. Other information of importance includes whether or not you are still menstruating and if so, whether your menstrual periods are regular or irregular. It should also be mentioned to the physician whether you have had a tubal ligation or complete or partial hysterectomy. Whether or not a patient is on hormone replacement pills, oral contraceptives (a.k.a. birth control pills), or medications for treatment of osteoporosis is relevant as well. Health maintenance issues such as dates of last Pap smear and last mammogram (and their results) are also relevant pieces of information. Additionally, a very important bit of information for the PCP, particularly on the first office visit is whether or not any of your close family members have had breast cancer.

Another area of importance with regard to optimizing the first office visit is the relevant family history. The relatives of greatest importance are your parents, grandparents, and siblings. In the event that you are adopted, family history must be obtained from the blood relatives to be valid. If their information is unobtainable, there is no need to worry. The most relevant information from the family history concerns those illnesses which have a hereditary pattern. How do you know which illnesses are hereditary? This is a difficult question to answer, as this area is so incredibly broad. However, if a certain disease is prominent in a family, regardless of what it is, it is still worth mentioning. Otherwise, due to it being the leading cause of death in the United States, it is very important to provide any information on what relations have had a history of heart disease, such as previous heart attacks, congestive heart failure, or arrhythmias, as well as strokes or any history of full-or partial-limb amputations resulting from poor circulation (from peripheral arterial or peripheral vascular disease).

Also of importance is whether or not you have any known drug allergies. An allergic response is often confused with an adverse reaction, and it is helpful to know the difference between the two. An allergic response can be mild or more severe. A mild response could be a minor skin rash. More severe reactions include the swelling of the face and wheezing and shortness of breath. One of the most severe allergic reactions, anaphylaxis, is a skin rash which makes the skin appear scalded and slough off the body. Adverse reactions, on the other hand, are less severe and are not life-threatening such as nausea, vomiting, diarrhea, headaches, and metallic taste. The important point is to be certain to convey your information to the doctor on the first visit. Of great importance to the physician as well is your social background. The most important information for the physician to know includes the following:

- Your marital status
- Whether you are employed, and if so, the type of work that you do
- Whether or not you are attending school
- Whether or not one is you are disabled, and if so, the reason(s) for disability
- Your social history, including whether or not you have children, grandchildren, or even great-grandchildren

- Your background, such as place of birth or where you were raised or grew up

Some aspects pertaining to social history can be quite personal, but it is very important that you be honest and up-front with the doctor regarding this area. This area of information includes whether or not you have a history of tobacco, alcohol or drug use, or any history of sexually transmitted diseases. Your sexual preference is important as well. Health-related issues such as having had a history of hepatitis, hepatitis C, tuberculosis, or what your HIV/AIDS status is are extremely important to convey to the physician as well. Lastly, any history of having received blood transfusions in the past is very important.

In summary, it is crucial that you obtain the optimal benefit from a doctor visit. The helpful hints offered in this chapter which can make this possible are as follows:

- Call the doctor's office in advance to see if actions such as having lab work done prior to the visit or being in a fasting state are necessary.

- Bring a list of your medications with the doses and schedules and/or the actual prescription bottles.

- Write down a problem list and bring it to the office visit but remember not to make it too overbearing for a single appointment. List the most important problems accordingly in order.

- Have available the names and telephone numbers of other physicians also involved in your management as a patient.

- Bring, if possible, copies of the results from previous studies, such as lab work, EKGs, and operative reports.

- Sign a release authorizing the new physician to obtain old records from a previous physician.

- Provide an accurate description of ongoing symptoms in as great detail as possible.

- Be able to provide as complete and accurate a history of the present illness as possible, as well as past medical history, OB/GYN history, and family history, allergies to medications, medication lists, and detailed aspects of your social history.

With the above information, you will optimize the benefits of your doctor visits which will further your ability to take charge of your health.

CHAPTER FIVE

PREVENTIVE MEDICINE

When reflecting upon your health, you often begin to realize how crucial a role it plays in determining your quality of life. Though quality of life may have many definitions to many of us, there is minimal doubt that if you are not in good health, your quality of life will not be at its optimal level. Oftentimes, you may take the quality of life issue for granted; allowing it to surface only when your health suddenly becomes compromised. This is usually a time for a serious re-evaluation and reordering of priorities–a time when life forces you to interrupt your hectic pace, which itself often leaves little time to reflect upon the aspects of life that are most important. When reflecting upon quality of life, you may begin to ask yourself if there were any measures that could have been taken which may have left you in better health today. In search of answers to this question, the concept of preventive medicine may very well come to the surface. It is safe to say that the best way to treat any disease state is to prevent it from happening in the first place. Although prevention is not always possible in the medical field, there are times when preventive measures save lives.

Upon establishing that preventive medicine has the objective of saving lives, before going any further with that thought, a moment should be taken to take a closer look at what the meaning or purpose of "saving lives" encompasses. The concept of saving lives is not always as clear-cut as it may sound. For example, taking measures which are aggressive to prolong the life of a 95-year-old person who has had several strokes, is no longer communicable, and is bed-bound with no chance of improvement is not the same as taking aggressive measures to save a 40-year-old, previously healthy person who has suffered a hemorrhagic stroke resulting from a cerebral aneurysm. The important point to be taken here is that in reality, the degree of aggressiveness of measures taken is determined by the situation at hand. With that being said, there are many appropriate situations where aggressive measures can be taken to both prevent and to treat disease states. The focus of preventive medicine is to identify those individuals who are at risk, and implement measures for early detection, which in turn, optimize more favorable outcomes.

Before beginning a discussion on the subject of preventive medicine, it is often helpful to have a clear and concise idea as to where preventive medicine fits into the big picture. Two very basic questions you may ask yourself are, "How is quality of life defined, and how is quality of life optimized?" Though quality of life may be defined in many ways to many individuals, the basic nuts-and-bolts definition is likely the same. Quality of life as I have defined it is "A state in which a reasonable degree of happiness can exist with a tolerable degree of discomfort." So therefore, quality of life can be enhanced by either increasing the degree of happiness or by decreasing the degree of discomfort. With reference to your health, enhancement of your quality of life is achieved through minimizing discomfort brought about by disease. Additionally, it can also be argued that by minimizing discomfort brought about by disease states, you will indirectly enhance happiness. Therefore, enhancing your quality of life by optimizing your health will have a two-fold effect. This is a wonderful revelation as it sets the stage for preventive medicine to become a vehicle by which the quality of life issue can be greatly enhanced. This revelation about the role of optimal health reveals the "cornerstone of the practice of modern day medicine." For the purpose of diet, exercise, prescription medications, surgeries, chemotherapies, and most other medical procedures is ultimately to optimize the state of happiness and to minimize discomfort.

One other objective in medicine is to prolong life. This objective of prolonging life, however, is not always straightforward. Prolonging life is not considered meaningful in all cases. Physicians are often faced with the dilemma of whether or not a situation in which one may be able to prolong life through a certain intervention will ultimately prolong life or merely prolong suffering. Such a case can be illustrated by the example of the ninety-five-year-old person who has had two strokes, which have rendered him non-communicative and bed-bound. The placement of a feeding tube would prolong his life. The question is now, by placing a feeding tube, is life and quality of life being prolonged or just merely life without a quality of life being prolonged? One way to help answer this question is to reflect back upon the definition of quality of life which is "a state in which a reasonable degree of happiness can exist with a minimal amount of discomfort." Therefore, the question that should be asked in this important decision is if this ninety-five-year-old person, who is non-communicative and bed-bound, is living with a reasonable degree of happiness and a tolerable degree of discomfort.

This same question can be asked when deciding whether or not to exercise aggressive measures such as brain decompressive surgery to save the life of the forty-year-old who has suddenly collapsed after suffering a brain hemorrhage resulting from a ruptured arterial aneurysm.

These two cases illustrate the two conditions which need to coexist in order to achieve success when exercising certain measures to optimize health. These two conditions are (1) to prolong life; and 2) to maintain or to enhance quality of life. Upon establishing a clear definition of your objective, it is clear that preventive medicine has its appropriate place and time. The next step is to determine how preventive medicine can be implemented. We have already established in previous chapters the most common causes of morbidity and mortality in the United States. At the top of the list, again, is cardiovascular disease, which accounts for approximately 1 million deaths per year. The second most common cause of death is cancer, which claims over half a million lives per year in the United States. Others on the list include chronic lower respiratory disease, diabetes, influenza, and motor vehicle accidents. With the determination of the most common causes of death, a method of identifying those at risk for morbidity and mortality resulting from these diseases must be obtained and implemented. Through countless clinical trials, risk factors for cardiovascular disease have been determined. Methods for identifying these individuals must be implemented so that preventive measures can then be taken with the objective of reducing morbidity and mortality. The risk factors identified as being associated with increased morbidity and mortality from cardiovascular disease are hypertension, diabetes, high cholesterol, smoking, a family history of the disease, being of the male gender or being a post-menopausal female, a sedentary lifestyle, increasing age (greater than 55 years) and others.

Upon identifying the risk factors for cardiovascular disease, the next step is to implement ways to control the risk factors. To begin with, uncontrolled hypertension, which is associated with an estimated 370,000 deaths from cardiovascular disease per year, can be controlled by methods such as diet, exercise, and the taking of prescription medications. Numerous clinical trials have shown huge reductions in morbidity and mortality when hypertension is controlled.

Diabetes mellitus continues to be on the rise, particularly in Hispanic children in the United States. Diabetes mellitus, particularly type two (which is by far the most common), is associated with atherosclerotic disease. This association between diabetes types one and two and atherosclerosis results in multiple systemic manifestations, such as diabetic-associated retinopathy (eye involvement), nephropathy (kidney involvement), as well as peripheral neuropathy (nerve involvement). Early identification of the disease is key. One warning sign is the presence of acanthosis nigricans, a darkened, velvet-like skin that, when found in children, increases their risk for developing diabetes. Regular doctor appointments with lab testing can also identify those at risk for diabetes mellitus. Those individuals with a positive family history should inform their physician so as to provide the proper screening tests such as a glucose tolerance test or a hemoglobin A1-c study. Like hypertension, diabetes mellitus can be controlled with diet, exercise, and prescription medications. Controlling diabetes has, like hypertension, been associated with marked reductions in morbidity and mortality through the numerous clinical trials.

High cholesterol, also referred to as hyperlipidemia or dyslipidemia, has been identified as a major risk factor for cardiovascular disease. An estimated 350,000 deaths per year from cardiovascular disease have been the result of uncontrolled cholesterol. Those with high cholesterol can be identified through blood tests. It is worth mentioning that cholesterol disorders come in different forms. The more precise term for high cholesterol is dyslipidemia. Cholesterol has several components which can be summed up in two basic categories: the good component (high-density lipoprotein or HDL) and the bad component (low-density lipoprotein or LDL). Those at risk for cardiovascular morbidity and mortality are those with both low good cholesterol (HDL) and high bad cholesterol (LDL). An easier way to remember which cholesterol is good and which is bad is thinking of the "H" in HDL as representing "hero" and the "L" in LDL representing "lowlife." Numerous clinical trials have revealed that control of dyslipidemia has also been associated with marked reductions in the morbidity and mortality that result from cardiovascular disease. Once again, like hypertension and diabetes, dyslipidemia can be controlled through diet, exercise, and prescription medications.

There is little more to be said about smoking that has not already been said, although it is worth mentioning again that smoking not only has a strong association with cardiovascular morbidity and mortality, but also with lung diseases such as lung cancer, chronic obstructive pulmonary disease, and emphysema. The only method for reducing morbidity and mortality from smoking is to stop smoking!

Family history of cardiovascular disease is very important and can be helpful in identifying those at risk for cardiovascular disease. A positive family history should make you more vigilant, and insist on a stress test when appropriate. It is important to notify your physician of a positive family history so that it is recorded in your history.

Males tend to be at higher risk than females for cardiovascular disease until menopause in women. This should increase vigilance and encourage these individuals to see their PCP at least once a year or more frequently if appropriate for management of other illnesses.

Post-menopausal women are at the same risk for cardiovascular disease as men. This risk can be lessened via hormone replacement therapy although, due to increased risk for endometrial (uterine) and breast cancer, the use of hormonal replacement therapy has been markedly decreasing.

Those with sedentary lifestyles have long been identified as having an increased risk of cardiovascular disease. It is advisable to exercise regularly although before engaging in an exercise regimen, should you be a candidate, it should be cleared by your PCP and cardiologist, possibly via a stress test if your PCP recommends it, prior to beginning an exercise program.

Aging, in and of itself, is a risk factor for cardiovascular disease. Although there are no treatments for age, realizing that age is a risk factor should prompt you to schedule and attend regular office visits with your PCP, diet and exercise if possible, and take prescribed medications regularly.

Cancer is the second-leading cause of death in the United States today. Cancer accounts for over 500,000 deaths per year. Like cardiovascular disease, there needs to be a method of identifying those at risk in order to implement early interventions which will allow for an optimal outcome, in turn, reducing morbidity and mortality. Again, the best treatment of a disease is prevention. Two factors need to be taken into account when exercising prevention. Firstly, the most commonly occurring cancer types need to be identified, and secondly, those cancers which have available screening tools must also be identified. When these two factors are accounted for, the appropriate measures can then be implemented. For example, it is imperative that women follow the recommendations for regular Pap smears outlined by the College of Gynecology and the American Cancer Society for the prevention of cervical cancer. The same applies to mammograms for the detection of breast cancer. As for colon cancer, the detection methods of hemoccult studies, flexible sigmoidoscopy, barium enemas, and colonoscopy are to be followed as per recommendation by the College of Gastroenterology and the American Cancer Society. Lastly, for prostate cancers, guidelines as per the College of Urology and the American Cancer Society call for the performance of digital rectal exams and annual PSA level checkups in order to screen for this cancer.

In summary, when looking at the big picture, the best treatment for a disease is prevention. The leading causes of morbidity and mortality as identified by the appropriate agencies need to be identified so as to make the largest impact possible on disease states. It is also important to remember that the purpose of reducing morbidity and mortality is to prolong the length and quality of life. The optimizing of quality of life is a prerequisite for exercising preventive medicine. It is with this clear view of the big picture that preventive medicine can find its appropriate place in helping you to take charge of your health.

CHAPTER SIX

HEALTH-CARE ISSUES FOR AGES 25–40

Reaching the age of twenty-five years is an accomplishment in and of itself. Reaching it means you have survived the difficult teenage years and early twenties, which years were, for most, a period of discovery, learning hard lessons, and heavy-duty emotional growth through experience. The ages of twenty-five to forty represent a period in which the core of your life may be defined. Permanent milestones like getting married, starting a family, and getting a steady job may be initiated in this age period. In other words, you will most likely accomplish what is often referred to as "settling down."

For some, the ages of twenty-five to forty may be different. For example, if you are a late bloomer, for different reasons, you may still be involved in an intense active pursuit of a college graduate, or post-graduate degree. You may also be investing a great deal of effort and time in your current career in an effort to improve your status and income.

The period of twenty-five to forty years, in terms of health, represents a unique period. Often, this is a period in which your life has earned a certain degree of wisdom resulting from surviving the teens and early twenties. This degree of wisdom is combined with a period of generally good health allowing you to make quantum leaps of progress in life. This unique period may allow you to lay a solid foundation for the later years in your life in which "the spirit may be willing, but the flesh may be weak."

Let there be no mistake that these accomplishments that you make in an effort to improve yourself, either for your own personal benefit or for the benefit of your family or other loved ones, are the result of being self-motivated with the necessary discipline to carry out these goals. This self-motivation and discipline will only be achieved through persistent effort. As always, there may be exceptions to these rules.

Living in a world where goals are achieved through effort and character-building, the ages of twenty-five to forty represent a time in which you can lay the groundwork for the later years. One of the reasons that you are able to accomplish so much during this period is that in general, you are blessed with good health which allows for higher levels of mental, physical, and emotional stress tolerance. This period may very well be the "honeymoon period." The honeymoon period is the period when you may enjoy good health with minimal effort exerted—when you are in the pre-hypertensive, pre-diabetic, pre-high cholesterol, pre-cardiovascular or pre-cancerous state. This is a time in which these diseases may remain "under the radar."

In an effort to fend off or to delay this "pre-morbid state" it is important to identify those risk factors during this particular age period. For the individuals in the 25–40 age range, the leading causes of death are, in order:

1. Motor vehicle accidents

2. Cancer

3. Cardiovascular disease

4. Suicide and homicide

In reference to motor vehicle accidents, morbidity and mortality can often be reduced through efforts as simple as exercising common sense and good driving habits. For starters, you must make sure to fasten your seat belt—not only because it is the law, but because it saves lives! Your chances of surviving a motor vehicle accident are greater if you are wearing a seatbelt than if you are not! Additionally, you should practice defensive driving. You should never assume that the other driver is going to practice safe driving habits. The mixture of drinking and driving is a combination that has proven deadly from day one. Alcohol-related motor vehicle accidents have claimed the lives of so many, and the irony is that the inebriated individual usually walks away with minimal, if any, injuries. All parties lose in the event of a fatal motor vehicle accident—the victims, the families, and loved ones, as well as the culprits and their families who have to live with the aftermath for the rest of their lives. So, the bottom line is, buckle up, practice defensive driving, don't drink and drive, don't drive while tired, and use common sense!

Another leading cause of death between 25 and 40 is cancer. Although not all cancers are detectable or curable, it is important to focus on the cancers which can be detected. For women, a detectable cancer during ages 25–40 is cervical cancer. Early detection can be made via Pap smear. Pap smears should begin three years after becoming sexually active, and no later than age 21. Risk factors for cervical cancer include human papilloma virus (HPV). (Pap smear is discussed in greater detail in Chapter 8.)

In men, testicular cancer most commonly occurs in the age bracket of 25–40. Early detection is the key. Early detection can be accomplished by physically examining the testes in much the same way a self-breast examination is performed for early detection of breast cancer. The presence of a scrotal mass should prompt an immediate visit to the primary care physician. A sonogram of the scrotum is usually ordered to distinguish between a cystic (fluid-filled) mass and a solid mass. If the mass is solid, a referral to a urologist should be the next step in order so as to perform further testing to make a diagnosis.

Breast cancer screening may be done in this age range of 25–40 in patients who have first-degree family members with a history of breast cancer—particularly if the breast cancer was diagnosed before the age of 50 years. The screening method of choice is the mammogram. A sonogram is not a diagnostic tool, but rather a study which distinguishes between a cystic or fluid-filled lesion and a solid mass lesion. The sonogram may be used when a mass is felt on physical exam or to clarify abnormal or suspicious mammography findings. If solid, the lesion is usually biopsied. Of note, men can also get breast cancer although not as common as women. For men, it is advisable to be tested with mammography and sonography when symptomatic. (For more details, mammography is discussed in greater detail in Chapter 8.)

Prostate cancer, although rarely seen in the age bracket of 25–40 years, should be mentioned. The signs and symptoms of prostate cancer may be urinary frequency or urgency, loss of bladder control, back pain, and/or urinary hesitancy. These symptoms are not specific to prostate cancer, but their presence should raise the suspicion for prostate cancer. The prostate-specific antigen study (PSA) is also a helpful screening study for detection of prostate cancer.

Colorectal cancer is another malignancy rarely seen in the 25–40 years age bracket. Those at risk are individuals who have first-degree relatives diagnosed with colorectal cancer before the age of 60. A number of screening studies are available for colorectal cancer. Hemoccult testing, where several stool samples are examined for occult blood (blood which is not visible to the naked eye) are the least invasive and the least expensive. Unfortunately, hemoccult testing is also the least specific study. Other studies for stool DNA are available which are more sensitive and specific. These stool DNA studies are only offered through certain labs. Other studies for colorectal cancer screening are the flexible sigmoidoscopy, double contrast air barium enema, and the colonoscopy. The colonoscopy is the gold standard for colorectal cancer screening. For further details, more on colorectal cancer screening appears in Chapter 8.

Cardiovascular disease needs no introduction, as it is by far the leading cause of death in the United States. Those individuals at risk for cardiovascular events—particularly heart attack, stroke, congestive heart failure, and peripheral vascular arterial disease—are those with risk factors such as heredity, hypertension, dyslipidemia, diabetes, tobacco use, proteinuria, and sedentary lifestyle. It is imperative that those diagnosed with these diseases or conditions be identified so that preventive measures can be taken. These preventive measures include a proper diet, exercise, control of hypertension, dyslipidemia, diabetes, and proteinuria, and the cessation of smoking.

The power of diet and exercise cannot be emphasized enough. The discussion about diet is endless although the key factors are basic which are the presence of: 1) nutrient balance, and 2) calorie quantity appropriateness. This basically leaves out crash diets and fad diets for the most part as these types of diets often either lack sufficient nutrients or have calorie counts which are either too high or too low. Exercise is also of great importance and recommendations are thirty minutes of cardiovascular (aerobic) daily although this may vary depending on overall health and age. For best recommendations, discuss with your primary care physician what level of activity would be most appropriate for you as clearance for example from a cardiologist or a pulmonologist may be indicated prior to beginning an exercise program. The end result of a proper diet in combination with exercise can, at times, abolish or markedly reduce the need for medication. Regular exercise can have a very positive effect on cardiovascular health when medically cleared by your physician and when recommended levels of activity are followed.

Hypertension is more prevalent now than ever—particularly in women. The most recent guidelines for management of hypertension are more aggressive than ever before. Clinical trials continue to demonstrate that for hypertension, lower (systolic blood pressure below 120mm hg) is better. The current guidelines for hypertension are less than 140/90 mmHg. Briefly, systolic blood pressure represents the pressure within the heart during its contractile (squeezing) phase and the diastolic blood pressure represents the pressure within the heart during the relaxation (dilated) phase. If a patient is diabetic or suffers from kidney disease, the goals for blood pressure are less than 130/80. As of 2003, a new category called "pre-hypertension" exists which includes those individuals with an SBP (systolic blood pressure) of 120 to 140 mmHg and a DBP (diastolic blood pressure) of 80 to 90 mmHg. At the time of printing, there are approximately 65 million hypertensives in the United States, of which 29 million are men and 36 million are women. At the age of approximately 50 years, women surpass men in prevalence of hypertension. If the number of pre-hypertensives were added to the number of hypertensive patients, the total would be approximately 100 million individuals. In the United States, approximately 1 million people die each year from cardiovascular disease. As was mentioned in a previous chapter, it is believed that approximately 370,000 out of these 1 million individuals have cardiovascular events resulting from uncontrolled hypertension. It is with these facts in mind that the importance of controlling blood pressure is illustrated.

A positive family history of cardiovascular disease is a strong risk factor for cardiovascular events. Therefore, if you have close family members with known cardiovascular disease, this should prompt you to see a primary care physician to screen for other risk factors as well, such as diabetes, hypertension, dyslipidemia, and proteinuria. These doctor visits will minimize morbidity and mortality through early identification, particularly if you have a strong family history of cardiovascular disease. A strong family history will likely prompt a physician to be more aggressive in evaluating and treating you.

Diabetes mellitus is an enormous risk factor for cardiovascular disease. There are very few organ systems, if any, that diabetes does not adversely affect. Many diabetics are almost certain to die from a cardiovascular event. Diabetes is the sixth-leading cause of death in the U.S. In the year 2002, diabetes resulted in over 73,000 deaths. Diabetes is strongly associated with atherosclerosis, which in turn increases the risk for heart attack, stroke, kidney disease, and diabetic retinopathy. Screening for diabetes can be performed primarily through laboratory blood studies. Screening can be as simple as the performance of a random (within five hours of most recent food ingestion) blood/ serum glucose level test or a two-hour post-prandial (after eating) blood glucose level test. The most common blood test for diabetes assessment is the hemoglobin A_{1C} (also known as the glycohemoglobin). The hemoglobin A_{1C} is routinely done on diabetics approximately every four months. But, for non-diabetics, it is not routinely done. A hemoglobin A_{1C} is usually performed if a random glucose level is found to be elevated, if glucose is found on a urinalysis, or if a patient has clinical signs of diabetes, such as frequent thirst, hunger, and/or urinary frequency. Tight control of diabetes has been shown to result in statistically significant reductions in cardiovascular events. The current target of diabetes is a hemoglobin A_{1C} of less than or equal to 6.5%.

Dyslipidemia, also known as hyperlipidemia or high cholesterol, is probably the most common new diagnosis made in a primary care physician's office. Of the approximately 1 million deaths in the United States resulting from cardiovascular disease, approximately 350,000 of them are believed to be in part a result of uncontrolled dyslipidemia. A great deal of research has been done in this area via clinical trials. There is strong evidence which demonstrates that tight control of the bad cholesterol—a.k.a. LDL or low-density lipoprotein—is associated with marked reductions in the risk for cardiovascular events. If an individual is at high risk for a cardiovascular event, recent guidelines suggest an LDL of less than 70. If an individual is at moderate risk, the suggested LDL level is less than 100. If an individual is at minimal risk, the recommended LDL level is less than 130. As for the good cholesterol—a.k.a. HDL or high-density lipoprotein—clinical trials suggest that for men, levels of greater than 40 and for women, levels greater than 50 are associated with statistically significant reductions in cardiovascular events. HDL is regarded by many medical experts as "cardioprotective." As for triglycerides, which are biochemical entities related to cholesterol and are molecules (units) consisting of a combination of a glycerol molecule and three fatty acids much more research has been done, particularly recently, upon their role in cardiovascular disease. Although the direct role of triglycerides in cardiovascular disease is not as clear as that of HDLs or LDLs, the effects of elevated triglyceride counts are, at the very least, indirect. Elevated triglyceride levels result in elevated free fatty acid levels as a result of the breakdown of the triglyceride molecule (as the triglyceride molecule contains one glycerol molecule and three fatty acids). The result of elevated free fatty acids is the interference with glucose metabolism or transport, leading to glucose intolerance which results in diabetes. Diabetes, as we know, is strongly associated with the atherosclerotic process leading to an increased risk for heart attack, stroke, kidney, and retinal disease. Triglyceride levels are best if kept below 150.

Tobacco use is clearly a no-brainer. With all of the negative publicity, it is not difficult to convince anyone of the numerous downsides of smoking. Tobacco use, whether via smoking or chewing, offers no advantages and is destructive in many ways. Tobacco use has a strong association with increased risk for heart disease, peripheral vascular disease, chronic obstructive pulmonary disease, emphysema, and numerous types of cancers.

The presence of protein in the urine—a.k.a. proteinuria—is a strong risk factor for cardiovascular disease. Proteinuria is also a marker for kidney disease in a diabetic. Although not known nearly as well as the other risk factors for cardiovascular disease, protein-uria, particularly in diabetics, is associated in both a quantitative and qualitative manner with cardiovascular disease. In other words, even the smallest amounts of proteinuria in diabetics carry a risk for cardiovascular events and/or disease, and the greater the degree of proteinuria, the greater the risk of cardiovascular events/disease.

A sedentary lifestyle is also associated with an increased risk for cardiovascular disease. Physical activity has an overall more positive effect on the metabolism than any single drug known. In and of itself, physical activity improves glucose and lipid metabolism. It also has a weight-loss promoting effect, particularly if combined with calorie-restriction diets. Exercise has a tendency to promote an overall improvement in lifestyle, as many individuals who regularly exercise tend to have healthier eating habits. Many individuals who lose weight while on extreme-type diets, such as low-carbohydrates, tend to only keep the weight off if they continue to exercise on a regular basis. Exercise provides not only metabolic and cardiovas-cular benefits but also is helpful for treatment of stress, for it is through exercise that endorphins (nature's antidepressants) such as hormones are released. It is at times possible to avoid the need for antidepressant use through engaging in a regular exercise program. Therefore, avoiding a sedentary lifestyle by engaging in a regular exercise program may result in an improvement in glucose and lipid (cholesterol) metabolism. Exercise promotes weight loss and a healthy lifestyle, which can act as an adjuvant in treatment of depression.

DR. MAROTTA'S PREVENTATIVE
ORGANIZER HEALTH CHECKLIST AGES 25–40

CHECK	Intervention Or Study	Recommendations	Date of Previous Study	Results	Goals/Targets	Follow up Due Date
	Blood Pressure	Check once a year unless diagnosed with hypertension; if so, at PCP's[1] discretion.			Less than 140/90 or if diabetic or with kidney disease less than 130/80	
	Cholesterol Profile	Check once a year; if diagnosed with high cholesterol, at discretion of PCP.			Less than 2 risk factors[2]—For cardiovascular disease—LDL<130;HDL>40 if male; HDL>50 if female. Greater than 2 risk factors—LDL<100; HDL>40 if male; HDL>50 if female	
	Blood sugar/ Blood glucose	Check once a year, or if diabetic, at discretion of PCP.			Fasting blood sugar[3] <127;Random blood sugar<180 Hgb A1-C ≤ 6.5%	
	Tobacco use	Stop ASAP			Reduce cardiovascular and pulmonary morbidity/mortality, as well as from lung cancer.	
	Seatbelt	Buckle up/click it for both driver and passenger.			Reduce motor vehicle accidents along with accompanying morbidity/mortality	
	Tetanus vaccine / booster	Every ten years			Prevention of infection from clostridium tetani bacteria (lockjaw).	
	Influenza vaccine	Check with PCP for necessity if you have lung disease, diabetes, or immune system compromise.			Prevention of morbidity/mortality from complications of or as a direct result of infection from influenza virus.	
	Colonoscopy	Check with PCP if you have a family history of colorectal cancer prior to age 60 yrs. or have polyps or inflammatory bowel disease.			Prevention of colorectal cancer. Early detection reduces morbidity / mortality and optimizes outcomes.	
	Mammogram	At age 40 or above; if positive family history, at discretion of gynecologist or PCP.			Prevention of breast cancer, early detection reduces morbidity/mortality and optimizes outcomes.	
	Pap smear	Begin when sexually active or no later than age 21 yrs. If after age 30, 3 consecutive negative Paps every 2 to 3 yrs.			Prevention of cervical cancer. Early detection reduces morbidity/mortality and optimizes outcomes.	

PSA level	Begin PSA blood4 test at age 50 or sooner if symptoms present or at PCP's discretion.		Prevention of prostate cancer. Early detection reduces morbidity/mortality and optimizes outcomes.
Vision examination	Yearly if diabetic by ophthalmologist or at discretion of PCP.		Optimize vision/quality of life; prevent accidents due to poor vision.
Dental examination	Daily flossing / regular brushing. If symptomatic, at discretion of dentist.		Optimize dentition; improve quality of life.
Hearing examination	If symptomatic, see an ENT or audiologist		Prevent accidents due to poor hearing; optimize quality of life.

FOOT NOTES

1) PCP—Primary Care Physician

2) Regarding NCEP guidelines, risk factors for cardiovascular disease include hypertension, diabetes, high cholesterol, smoking, sedentary lifestyle, family history, microalbuminuria.

NCEP guidelines for diabetics or those with a history of a heart attack or stroke are as follows:

HDL of > 40 if male   HDL>50 if female   LDL of < 70   Triglycerides of < 150

3) Diabetes testing can be done with:

a) random glucose level

b) glucose tolerance test

c) Hgb A1-C.

4) PSA—Prostate Specific Antigen

CHAPTER SEVEN

HEALTH-CARE ISSUES FOR AGES 40–65

By the time you reach the ages between 40 and 65, the years of naivety have long since past. You have survived puberty, high school, and have possibly conquered the rigors of further education. You have generally settled on what will be your life-long vocation. You may have become a parent, and possibly even a grandparent. Reaching the age of 40 can be viewed in many ways. For some, the age of 40 represents a time in which the mind is mature enough to exercise wisdom in decision-making while, at the same time, you are as reasonably physically fit as when you were in your twenties. For others reaching the age of 40 represents a time in which you begin to experience the aches and pains of old injuries or arthritis which were not there when in your twenties or thirties. Also at 40 years, you may begin to realize that being over-weight, having hypertension, or diabetes is no longer something that just happens to other people—particularly "older people."

Regardless of how you may view reaching your forties, when it comes to health, you can no longer continue to rely on your youth to "bale you out." There are numerous reasons which explain how, at this age, people may begin to feel like they're starting to fall apart. For instance, at this point in time, you may be working longer hours to help make ends meet or to upgrade your standard of living. Working long hours can have a very negative effect on healthy living. By working long hours, you can get into a vicious cycle: You get home late and are too tired to exercise. You're also starving from a long, stressful day that left little time for a meal break. So you eat a heavy late meal which results in poor digestion and a great case of gastroesophageal reflux (a.k.a. heartburn). This cycle of not exercising and overeating usually results in weight gain and may also result in the development of hypertension, high cholesterol, and even diabetes. This results in a marked increase in the risk for cardiovascular disease.

Staying out of this cycle is not easy, as other factors exist which also may result in the "fat and unfit vicious cycle." For it may be at this same time that, if you are a parent, you may become very involved in your children's curricular and extracurricular activities which can be very time-and energy-consuming, again causing plans for diet and exercise to fall by the wayside. This "falling by the wayside" doesn't have to happen, although to prevent falling into the "fat and unfit vicious cycle," it will, without doubt, require effort, motivation, and discipline.

In establishing what the health concerns are between the ages of 40 and 65, the leading causes of mortality must be identified. These leading causes of death are as follows:

1. Cancer

2. Cardiovascular disease

3. Motor vehicle accidents

4. Suicide and homicide

5. Human immunodeficiency virus (HIV)

BREAST CANCER / MAMMOGRAPHY

At the age of 40, mammograms are recommended for all women. Mammograms may be recommended at an earlier age if there are close relatives that have been diagnosed with breast cancer. This is an issue that should be discussed with either the gynecologist or your PCP. The purpose of a mammogram is to detect breast cancer as early as possible. Early detection is of the essence, as a localized lesion has a 98% five-year survival rate as compared to a lesion with a localized spread which has a five-year survival rate of 81%. If breast cancer has had a diffuse spread (also known as metastasis) to other organs such as the lungs, brain, or liver, the five-year survival rate drops to 26%! The mammogram, as compared to clinical breast examination, offers the advantage of identifying lesions too small to be felt by the patient or the examiner. This may lead to earlier detection which improves the five-year survival rate.

A mammogram is essentially an X-ray of the breast. Technique is important. Therefore, it is optimal to have the mammogram performed by an experienced and qualified technician. Correct interpretation of the mammogram also requires a skilled radiologist. Therefore, it is optimal to have a mammogram performed at a location where competent technicians and radiologists are available. The skilled radiologist looks for calcifications in the breast X-ray and their characteristic patterns which suggest either a benign or a malignant diagnosis. Anyone who has had a mammogram will not argue the fact that they are uncomfortable. However, for optimal mammography, compression of the breast may be uncomfortable, but it is also of the utmost importance. It is very important to remember that mammograms do not detect all breast cancers. In spite of the fact that the mammogram is the most sensitive screening method, efforts must be made to optimize screening.

One of the ways to optimize the sensitivity of screening for breast cancer is to combine the self-breast or clinical breast examination findings with the mammogram findings. There may be instances where the self or clinical breast examination detects an abnormality which is not seen on mammography. If such is the case, a biopsy may next be performed which clarifies the diagnosis as either benign or malignant. The important point here is to realize that by combining both mammographic findings with clinical findings; the sensitivity of the screening technique is enhanced, resulting in earlier detection and better outcomes.

Women should learn to perform self-breast examinations and to use the best technique possible. Self-breast examinations should be performed approximately once a month and a clinical breast examination by the physician should be performed approximately once a year.

With regards to the self-breast examination, the patient needs first to inspect the breasts. Pertinent findings include discoloration, retraction, scaliness, pain, swelling, or a discharge of the nipple. Other pertinent findings include dimpling of the skin on the chest wall, a mass on the breast, or scaliness/redness of the chest wall. Any of these pertinent findings noted should immediately be reported to the physician in order to expedite making a diagnosis. Palpation of the breasts in search of masses is also important. Palpation technique should be learned from a qualified health-care professional. The self-breast examination should be performed approximately once a month.

Another breast imaging study is the breast ultrasound (or sonogram). This study helps to distinguish between a cystic (fluid-filled) and a solid mass. This study is ordered at the discretion of the physician and is not a diagnostic study, although it helps to narrow the possible diagnosis by ruling out a solid mass as opposed to a cystic mass.

PAP SMEARS

As previously mentioned, Pap smears should be started three years after becoming sexually active, and no later than age 21. At the age of 40, Pap smears are still recommended every year. There are exceptions to this rule. According to guidelines as per the American Cancer Society and the American College of Obstetrics and Gynecology, Pap smears should be performed yearly until the age of 30, at which time, if the three previous consecutive Pap smears have been normal, the Pap smear can be done every two to three years. According to guidelines by the U.S. Preventive Task Force in 2003, a Pap smear is recommended every three years, as according to their findings, there is no evidence to suggest that every year is better than every three years.

It is important to know that the Pap smear is a screening study performed to provide early detection of cervical cancer. The Pap smear is not a screening tool for cancers of the ovaries, uterus, or vagina. No screening studies exist for these cancers, although a blood test called a CA-125 can be helpful in diagnosing ovarian cancer. The gynecologist or primary care physician's role in the performance of a pelvic examination is of extreme importance as an addition to the Pap smear, as it may identify other diseases or malignancies. It is extremely important to report symptoms to the physician, such as vaginal bleeding, changes in the patterns of your menstrual cycles, or any pelvic pain, for example. Other important symptoms, such as the discovery of any skin lesions in the pelvic region, vaginal discharge, or pain upon urination, should be conveyed to your physician.

Close surveillance is never a bad idea, as the benefits which combine the Pap smear, pelvic examinations, and reported symptoms can only help in identifying problems, particularly those which have no screening studies such as vaginal, uterine, and ovarian cancers, and any other non-malignant diseases as well.

Another risk factor for cervical cancer is Human Papilloma Virus. Although HPV causes the majority of all cervical cancers, it rarely actually becomes cancerous. HPV usually resolves itself on its own. There are numerous serotypes of HPV. Certain serotypes have higher malignancy rates than others.

OSTEOPOROSIS / DEXA SCAN

Osteoporosis is a concern in the U.S. for both men and women. Osteoporosis can be defined as a pathological process resulting in the deterioration of bone density. This pathological process is essentially the result of an imbalance between bone building and bone destruction—more in favor of bone destruction. The disease essentially reduces bone density which results in a higher likelihood of bone fractures. The World Health Organization defines a bone mineral density of more than 2.5 standard deviations below the mean for a healthy adult woman. Osteopenia, or "near osteoporosis" is where bone mineral density is between 1.0 and 2.5 standard deviations below the mean for a healthy young adult woman.

Now that osteoporosis has been defined, the next step is to identify those at highest risk for it. In addition to low bodyweight, there are numerous risk factors for osteoporosis, most of which include:

- Post-menopausal woman not on hormone replacement therapy
- Age—particularly above 60 years
- Low testosterone levels/hypogonadism/male andropause
- Sedentary/low-activity lifestyle
- Non-African American ethnicity, especially Asian ethnicity
- Tobacco use
- Excessive alcohol use
- Excessive caffeine intake
- Low calcium or vitamin D intake
- Medications such as diuretics which result in calcium loss

The end result of osteoporosis is an increased risk for fractures, particularly of the vertebrae/spinal column and of the hip. Today, there are different types of treatments available for osteoporosis. These treatments consist of exercise and calcium supplementation as well as several types of prescription medications. For the optimal choice of prescription medication(s), consult your physician.

The study of choice to determine bone mineral density is the dual-energy X-ray absorptiometry also known as the DEXA scan. The recommendations regarding when and how often DEXA scans should be performed are not clear-cut before the age of 60.

However, in patients between ages 60 and 65 with multiple risk factors, routine screening is recommended. Once reaching the age of 65, routine screening is recommended to all. The frequency with which DEXA scans should be performed is not clear, although most health-care plans will cover a DEXA scan every two years or thereabouts.

It is noteworthy to mention that for males with low testosterone levels, a condition known as hypogonadism or male andropause, the risk for osteoporosis exists as it does in females, and a DEXA scan should also be considered.

COLORECTAL CANCER

Although for average-risk patients, colorectal cancer screening is not recommended until the age of 50, there will be indications for colorectal screening for patients in their forties, as well as patients who are younger than 40. Colorectal cancer is the fourth-leading cancer type and the second-leading cause of cancer deaths in the United States. Again, in an effort to minimize morbidity and mortality resulting from colorectal cancer, those at increased risk must be identified so as to optimize favorable outcomes. Those who are at increased risk at the age of 40 are the following:

- Those with first-degree relatives diagnosed before the age of 60
- Those with a history of adenomatous or villous polyps
- Those with a history of familial polyposis or of hereditary non-polyposis
- Those with a history of inflammatory bowel disease, such as ulcerative colitis or Crohn's disease

There are several available screening tools for colorectal cancer. Fecal occult blood testing is the least invasive and the least expensive. In this study, the patient is given three cards in which a stool specimen is collected and is sent to the lab to test for the presence of blood which is not visible to the naked eye. The disadvantage of this study is that it is not very specific, therefore, there will be a large number of false-positives. Fecal occult blood testing in high-risk patients is recommended once a year.

Another screening study for colorectal cancer is the flexible sigmoidoscopy. The advantage to this study is that it can be performed in the doctor's office and that it does not require sedation. The disadvantages to this study are that it is uncomfortable and that it visualizes only the distal part of the colon (although it is a fact that 80% of colorectal cancers arise in this same distal portion of the colon). What this means is that most cancers will be visualized with the flexible sigmoidoscopy, but a portion of them which occur in the more proximal portion of the colon will be missed.

It has been advocated that combining both fecal occult blood testing and periodic flexible sigmoidoscopy may improve the sensitivity of the screening for colorectal cancer. This combination has not, as of yet, been proven to be superior to flexible sigmoidoscopy alone.

A third screening study for colorectal cancer is the double air-contrast barium enema. This study has a high sensitivity and specificity, although in lesions of less than one centimeter, the sensitivity is markedly reduced. One advantage over the colonoscopy is that it does not require sedation, and one advantage of the double air-contrast barium enema over the flexible sigmoidoscopy is that it views the entire colon as opposed to only the distal portion.

The fourth screening study for colorectal cancer is the colonoscopy. This could well be considered the "gold standard" for colorectal cancer screening. The colonoscopy is the most sensitive and specific screening study for colorectal cancer, as well as for numerous other disorders of the colon. The colonoscopy offers the advantages of viewing the entire colon, unlike the flexible sigmoidoscopy which views only a portion of the colon. The colonoscopy, unlike the double contrast barium enema, offers the option of performing biopsies on suspicious lesions, as well as removal of lesions such as polyps if necessary. Unlike fecal occult testing, it offers a much greater degree of specificity. The colonoscopy, like other studies, also has risks involved, such as bleeding upon removal of lesions, bowel perforation, and the use of anesthesia/sedation. One added benefit of the colonoscopy is the fact that if the study results are normal, it is usually good for ten years.

PROSTATE CANCER

Although screening for prostate cancer is not indicated until the age of 50, there are rare cases which have occurred that are worth mentioning. What you should know with regard to prosate cancer is that the presence of signs and symptoms such as increased urinary frequency, loss of urinary continence, blood in the urine, pain on urination, and back pain, is the key to raising the physician's suspicion for prostate cancer. Additionally, having had a family history of prostate cancer at an early age should raise the suspicion of prostate cancer. Upon raising the suspicion, a digital rectal examination, PSA level (prostate-specific antigen), and a urology referral should be the next steps taken. The presence of the symptoms may indeed prompt a cystoscopy and prostate biopsy by the urologist in order to make the diagnosis.

CARDIOVASCULAR DISEASE

Cardiovascular disease, as mentioned, is the second-leading cause of mortality in this age range. It is imperative that those at greatest risk for cardiovascular disease be identified. Those at most risk are those who identify with one or more of the following qualities:

- Have hypertension
- Have dyslipidemia (a.k.a. high cholesterol)
- Have diabetes
- Use tobacco
- Lead a sedentary lifestyle
- Have a family history of cardiovascular disease
- Are over the age of 50
- Are a post-menopausal female
- Are of the male gender

For a fuller discussion of hypertension, the chapter for ages 25–40 offers a more detailed information section. That being said, in a more brief discussion, hypertension is strongly associated with age and with gender. At the age of 40 years, it is not uncommon for men and women alike to discover that they have hypertension. Hypertension is, more often than not, asymptomatic. Defined as having a blood pressure greater than 140/90 or in the case of diabetics or those with chronic kidney disease, as greater than 130/80 mmHg (millimeters of mercury), hypertension is a major risk factor for cardiovascular events, and as such, must be treated aggressively. Therefore an annual appointment with your primary care physician is recommended to allow for a prompt diagnosis and subsequent treatment. If you suffer from headaches, blurred vision, and/or dizziness, a blood pressure check is a good idea, even if it has been less than one year since you last saw your primary care physician.

The detection of dyslipidemia, or high cholesterol, is only possible through a blood test. This can be done on your annual visit to your primary care physician. Dyslipidemia is discussed also in the chapter for age ranges 25–40 years. Dyslipidemia is, like hypertension, a major risk factor for cardiovascular disease, and its early detection and treatment is of the utmost importance. For individuals with minimal other risk factors, the HDL in males is recommended at 40 or greater and HDL in females at 50 or greater. For individuals with minimal risk factors, the LDL is recommended at 130 or less according to the most recent guidelines. If an individual has more than two risk factors for cardiovascular disease, for example, hypertension, family history of heart disease, and age, the recommended LDL is 100 or less. Finally, for the individual who has had a previous cardiovascular event such as a heart attack or stroke, or who has diabetes mellitus, the recommended LDL is less than 70 according to the most recent guidelines.

Diabetes mellitus, which is also discussed in the 25–40 year old age range chapter, is an enormous risk factor for cardiovascular disease. Diabetes, in 2002, accounted directly for over 73,000 deaths. Diabetes is a disease which adversely affects virtually every organ system. Diabetes mellitus accounts for 20% of all health-care expenditures yearly, totaling over 130 billion dollars per year. There are currently over 20 million diabetics in the United States. A minimum of yearly screening through blood testing upon reaching the age of 40 years should help in making a diagnosis. It is believed that by the time an individual is diagnosed with diabetes type 2, that individual has been diabetic for approximately five years. Symptoms which suggest diabetes are the sudden onset of increased thirst, increased urination, and increased appetite. Those individuals with a family history of diabetes should be especially vigilant by having lab work done at least once yearly and being aware of the symptoms of diabetes. Upon being diagnosed with diabetes, it is very important to follow proper dietary practices as well as exercise if possible. Keeping regular doctor's appointments which are usually every four months is also important. Diabetics should have regular ophthalmology examinations every year in order to screen for diabetic-related retinopathy. Diabetics should be very aware of their vulnerability to foot problems as well. These foot problems are the result of the effect of the diabetes on the nervous system, which is called peripheral neuropathy. Peripheral neuropathy in diabetics results in a loss of feeling or sensation in the feet. As a result of this loss of feeling, for example, a diabetic may be cutting their foot on a small rock in their shoe and not even feel it. Therefore, exercising good foot hygiene is of utmost importance to a diabetic. If you are a diabetic, it is not a bad idea to have a checkup by a podiatrist and also to establish yourself with a podiatrist for that very reason.

Tobacco use, once again, offers no benefits to anyone. Tobacco use, unfortunately, is associated heavily with cardiovascular disease, as well as with pulmonary diseases such as chronic obstructive pulmonary disease (COPD), emphysema, and lung cancer. Therefore, it can be said that tobacco use contributes to the two top causes of death. Tobacco use not only exacerbates the risks for lung cancers, but also for many other types of cancer such as head, neck, and esophageal cancers. Whenever you smoke, it may affect other innocent bystanders who may be the victims of secondhand smoke inhalation. Even upon cessation of smoking, the increased risk for lung cancers remain for as long as twenty years! By quitting the use of tobacco, you are taking a major step towards reducing the risk of cardiovascular disease as well as the risk of contracting several forms of cancer additionally, it has been shown that quitting tobacco adds to one's lifetime regardless of when one quits and the earlier one quits the more years they add to their life. Leading a sedentary lifestyle increases the risk of cardiovascular disease. The benefits of diet, exercise, and achieving your ideal body weight cannot be emphasized enough. Exercise has a very favorable affect on your metabolism. You can eat with greater liberty when engaging in regular exercise. Exercise offers benefits not only to the cardiovascular system, but also to the pulmonary system. Individuals who lose substantial amounts of weight have a greater tendency to keep the weight off if they continue to engage in a regular exercise program. A regular exercise program, particularly if the exercise is aerobic in nature, results in a lower heart rate which results in more efficient cardiac function. In other words, less work for the heart in turn allows for a greater reserve in the event that the heart is stressed.

Family history of cardiovascular disease and certain types of malignancies are also risk factors for cardiovascular disease and certain cancers. It is important that you convey this information to the physician, as it may affect the timing of when screening studies are performed. For example, if you have a strong family history of cardiac disease, it may affect the degree of aggressiveness exercised by a cardiologist, such as whether he will do an exercise stress test versus a cardiac catheterization. Another example is a situation where a patient's first-degree relative was diagnosed with cancer before the age of 60. Instead of recommending colorectal cancer screening at the age of 50, colorectal cancer screening via colonoscopy may be recommended as early as the age of 30. These are two examples of where family history can be extremely important.

Age, in and of itself, is a risk factor for cardiovascular disease and cancer. At the age of 50, for example, even in patients without obvious risk factors for colorectal cancer, screening in men and women should still be performed. Also at the age of 50, in men, prostate cancer screening should be performed. Unfortunately, age is a risk factor for just about anything that is potentially harmful!

Women, until the time of menopause, are at lower risk for cardiovascular disease than men. This is likely due in part to the cardioprotective effects of estrogen. Additionally, at approximately the same time as menopause, more women develop hypertension than men up until the time of death.

DR. MAROTTA'S PREVENTATIVE
ORGANIZER HEALTH CHECKLIST AGES 40-65

CHECK	Intervention Or Study	Recommendations	Date of Previous Study	Results	Goals/Targets	Follow up Due Date
	Blood Pressure	Check once a year unless diagnosed with hypertension; if so, at PCP's[1] discretion.			Less than 140/90 or if diabetic or with kidney disease less than 130/80	
	Cholesterol Profile	Check once a year; if diagnosed with high cholesterol, at discretion of PCP.			Less than 2 risk factors[2]—for cardiovascular disease —LDL≤130 HDL>40 if male; HDL>50 if female. If greater than 2 risk factors, LDL<100;HDL>40 if male;HDL>50 if female.	
	Blood sugar/ Blood glucose	Check once a year with random serum glucose or if diagnosed with diabetes mellitus, at discretion of PCP. (ex. every 4 mos.)			Fasting blood glucose[3] <127 Random blood glucose <180 Hgb A1-C ≤ 6.5%	
	Tobacco use	Stop ASAP			Reduce cardiovascular and pulmonary disease, along with lung cancer	
	Seatbelt	Buckle up/click it for both driver and passenger.			Reduce motor vehicle accidents along with accompanying morbidity/mortality	
	Influenza vaccine	Check with PCP for necessity if you have lung disease, diabetes, or immune system compromise.			Prevention of morbidity / mortality from complications of or as a direct result of infection from influenza virus	
	Colonoscopy	Check with PCP if you have a family history of colorectal cancer prior to age 60 yrs. or have polyps, inflammatory bowel disease.			Prevention of colorectal cancer. Early detection reduces morbidity / mortality and optimizes outcomes.	
	Mammogram	At age 40 or above; if positive family history, at discretion of gynecologist or PCP(usually sooner)			Prevention of breast cancer, early detection reduces morbidity/mortality and optimizes outcomes.	
	Pap smear	Begin when sexually active or no later than age 21 yrs. If after age 30, 3 consecutive negative Paps every 2 to 3 yrs.			Prevention of cervical cancer. Early detection reduces morbidity/mortality and optimizes outcomes.	

Pap smear	Begin when sexually active or no later than age 21 yrs. If after age 30, 3 consecutive negative Paps every 2 to 3 yrs.	Prevention of cervical cancer. Early detection reduces morbidity/mortality and optimizes outcomes.
DEXA scan / bone densitometry	High risk begin at age 60; all female patients 65 and over.	Prevention and treatment[4] of osteoporosis. Early detection reduces chance of fractures.
PSA level	Begin PSA[5] blood test at age 50 or sooner if symptoms present or at PCP's discretion.	Prevention of prostate cancer. Early detection reduces morbidity/mortality and optimizes outcomes. PSA less than 4.0 or at discretion of PCP.
Vision examination	If symptomatic or at discretion of optometrist / ophthalmologist.	Optimize vision/quality of life; prevent accidents due to poor vision.
Dental examination	Daily flossing / regular brushing. Yearly checkup / cleaning or discretion of dentist.	Optimize dentition; improve quality of life.
Hearing examination	If symptomatic, see an ENT or audiologist	Optimize quality of life; prevent accidents resulting from poor hearing.

FOOT NOTES

1) PCP—Primary Care Physician
2) Regarding NCEP guidelines, risk factors for cardiovascular disease include hypertension, diabetes, high cholesterol, smoking, sedentary lifestyle, family history, microalbuminuria.
   NCEP guidelines for diabetics or those with a history of a heart attack or stroke are as follows:
   HDL of > 40 if male   HDL>50 if female   LDL of < 70   Triglycerides of < 150
3) Diabetes testing can be done with:
   a) random glucose level
   b) glucose tolerance test
   c) Hgb A1-C.
4) High risk for osteoporosis includes:
   a) post-menopausal state without hormone replacement therapy   f) excessive alcohol
   b) age over 60 years   g) excessive caffeine intake
   c) low-activity lifestyle   h) low calcium and vitamin D intake
   d) low body weight   i) medications
   e) tobacco use   j) low testosterone levels in males.
5) PSA—Prostate Specific Antigen

CHAPTER EIGHT

HEALTH-CARE ISSUES FOR AGES 65 AND OVER

Reaching the age of 65 years deserves some congratulations. For at age 65, it is safe to say that in the vast majority of cases, an individual has whatever accomplishments which define them in their rear-view mirror. In other words, whatever defines your life has, in the majority of cases, come and gone. So, does this mean that life ends at the age of 65? No way! For 65 or above can in a more mature way be viewed as a beginning of another chapter in your life. At this point, you should still continue to set goals especially if you remain in good health. By the mere fact that you have reached retirement age your past experiences and garnered wisdom will allow you to provide others of a younger age and less experience with a wealth of knowledge and guidance. This ability to help others can provide for you a great deal of satisfaction. It is this satisfaction at times which may be the sole driving force for many to get up every morning with great enthusiasm. For reaching the age of seniority, although different from your more youthful years, can among other aspects provide the opportunity for you to give back to others. This giving back may provide even greater satisfaction than receiving. This age range of 65 years and older may most clearly illustrate the meaning of the phrase, "It is far greater to give than to receive."

The idea of knowing that life can be just as interesting or even better at this age may also provide encouragement to those who are struggling at younger ages. Knowing that people in general are living longer these days can also be a motivation to take care of your health at younger ages in order to be in more optimal health later in life. The knowledge and wisdom acquired in your earlier years may well serve as the glue that keeps you together, particularly if you do have to deal with the health problems which may be encountered with old age. It is with the knowledge and wisdom acquired through years of experience that you will be able to view entering retirement age as the beginning of another stage in life which provides an opportunity to excel, rather than marking the end of "the good old days."

You must be realistic when reaching the age of 65 or above. It will require more attention and work to maintain your health as you age. By taking charge of your health through exercising good health maintenance, you will optimize the quality as well as the longevity of your life. Longevity with quality is the name of the game when it comes to health care.

In the pursuit of longevity with quality in the age range of 65 and above, as with the previous age ranges, the leading causes of death must be identified and measures taken to minimize them. Next, in identifying those at risk, measures must be taken to prevent or at least to minimize the occurrence of those factors which may predispose individuals to the leading causes of death, or more practically stated, the leading causes of morbidity and mortality.

The leading causes of death in the age range of 65 years and above are as follows:

1. Cardiovascular disease

2. Cancer

3. Chronic lower respiratory diseases

4. Diabetes mellitus

5. Influenza and pneumonia

Cardiovascular diseases include myocardial infarction (or heart attack), cerebrovascular accident (or stroke), congestive heart failure, and peripheral vascular diseases such as gangrene of the extremities. As a quick review, those at the most risk for cardiovascular disease are those who (1) have hypertension, (2) have diabetes mellitus, (3) have dyslipidemia (or high cholesterol), (4) have a family history of the disease, (5) use tobacco, (6) have proteinuria (or protein in the urine), (7) lead a sedentary lifestyle, (8) are post-menopausal, (9) are of the male gender, and (10) are 65 years old and above. For a more detailed discussion on risk factors for cardiovascular disease, see the previous two chapters regarding age ranges 25–40 years and 40–65 years.

The cancers for which screening studies are available are the following:

• Breast cancer via mammograms

• Cervical cancer via Pap smear

• Colorectal cancers via colonoscopy, flexible sigmoidoscopy, barium enema (double contrast), or fecal occult blood testing

- Prostate cancer via annual prostate-specific antigen and digital rectal examinations

These screening studies are discussed in greater detail in the previous chapters involving age ranges 25–40 years and 40–65 years.

Chronic lower respiratory diseases refer to those diseases which involve the lungs. The most common of the chronic diseases are chronic obstructive pulmonary disease (COPD), emphysema, asthma, and chronic bronchitis. Other types of chronic lower respiratory diseases are pulmonary fibrosis, asbestosis, cystic fibrosis, silicosis, berylliosis, and others. Although these diseases are not curable, measures can be taken to minimize their morbidity and mortality. The simplest illustration of minimizing the morbidity and mortality resulting from COPD/emphysema is to quit smoking, and to avoid becoming a victim of secondhand smoke inhalation. Another simple means of minimizing morbidity and mortality is to avoid exposure to causative agents like asbestos, silica in silicosis, and beryllium in berylliosis. With regard to asthma, it is important to identify the triggering agent, such as allergies, exercise, or change in weather. Upon being diagnosed with a chronic lower respiratory disease, it is important to be compliant with medications like inhalers, nebulizers, supplemental oxygen, as well as oral medications (medications by mouth). It is also very advisable to establish yourself with a pulmonologist. For those individuals with chronic pulmonary diseases, it is very advisable to receive the pneumonia and influenza vaccine on a regular basis as the ability to survive pneumococcal pneumonia and influenza is diminished due to compromised lung function.

Diabetes mellitus is also a leading cause of death in the elderly. As of today, no cure exists for diabetes, although major improvements in terms of minimizing morbidity and mortality have been made. Treatment consists of diet and exercise, oral medications, subcutaneous insulin injections and recently, inhaled insulin. Diabetes, by itself, is a leading cause of death and is also a major risk factor for cardiovascular disease. Diabetes mellitus is discussed in greater detail in both chapters regarding age ranges 25–40 and 40–60.

Influenza, (a.k.a. the flu), and pneumonia are leading causes of morbidity and mortality in the elderly. Although no absolute proof exists, aging, different theories suggest, adversely affects the immune system. With regard to pneumonia, when the cause is of bacterial origin, it can successfully be treated. However, even if pneumonia is of bacterial etiology, if treatment is not given before it spreads from the lungs into the bloodstream, it can be deadly. Influenza can also be deadly in the elderly. The complications of influenza are several. Examples include respiratory failure, dehydration with resultant electrolyte disturbances, and others. The bottom line is that if elderly patients are not aggressively treated when they contract either a pneumonia or influenza, the end result may be death. Influenza can be prevented by receiving the flu vaccine on a yearly basis. Additionally, if the flu is contracted, there are three oral medications available which are effective against influenza A which are amantadine, rimantadine, and oseltamivir. There are also two treatments which are effective against both influenza A and influenza B strains which are zanamivir and oseltamivir. Clinically, in terms of signs and symptoms, influenza

A and influenza B are indistinguishable, although influenza A is more common. The two strains A and B can be distinguished by testing secretions from the nose, throat, or mouth. One of the complications of influenza is that it can weaken the immune system, leaving it vulnerable to bacteria which can set in and cause a secondary infection which increases the likelihood of death, particularly in the elderly. The best way to reduce morbidity and mortality from pneumonia is through vaccination. The pneumonia vaccine should be received approximately every five to ten years. As concerning treatment, there are numerous antibiotics available if the cause is bacterial. Other causes of pneumonia include some viruses, such as herpes, fungi, and tuberculosis. Though these are all far less common than the bacterial pneumonia, viral influenza and parainfluenza, they are also treatable.

Other aspects of general health which have not been mentioned are dental health, vision, and hearing. Although there are no set ages for maintenance, you must use a common-sense approach in reference to dental health, vision, and hearing. With regard to dental health, it is helpful to become established with a dentist. Remembering both to keep regular appointments for teeth cleaning and to floss are very important. It is never a good idea to wait until a toothache becomes excruciating to present to the dentist, as a toothache is usually a signal that something is wrong. In reference to vision, it is also important to have regular eye exams. For those who are diabetic, it is important to see an ophthalmologist at least once a year to check for diabetic retinopathy. Other conditions, such as glaucoma, require more frequent visits. In reference to hearing, if a deficiency is apparent, a referral to an ear, nose, and throat specialist, a.k.a. an otorhinolaryngologist, is recommended, as certain hearing deficiencies may benefit from hearing devices. It is recommended, as in other areas of health maintenance, to make and keep regular appointments with your ear, nose, and throat specialist.

DR. MAROTTA'S PREVENTATIVE
ORGANIZER HEALTH CHECKLIST AGES 65 AND OVER

CHECK	Intervention Or Study	Recommendations	Date of Previous Study	Results	Goals/Targets	Follow up Due Date
	Blood Pressure	Check once a year unless diagnosed with hypertension; if so, at PCP's[1] discretion.			Less than 140/90 or if diabetic or with kidney disease less than 130/90	
	Cholesterol Profile	Check once a year; if diagnosed with high cholesterol, at discretion of PCP.			Less than 2 risk factors for cardiovascular disease[2] LDL≤130 HDL>40 if male; HDL>50 if female. Greater than 2 risk factors for cardiovascular disease, LDL<100; HDL>40 if male; HDL>50 if female.	
	Blood sugar/ Blood glucose	Check once a year with random serum glucose or if diagnosed with diabetes mellitus, at discretion of PCP. (ex. every 4 mos.)			Fasting blood glucose[3] <127 Random blood glucose <180 Hgb A1-C ≤ 6.5%	
	Tobacco use	Stop ASAP			Reduce cardiovascular and pulmonary disease, along with lung cancer	
	Seatbelt	Buckle up/click it for both driver and passenger.			Reduce motor vehicle accidents along with accompanying morbidity/mortality	
	Pneumonia vaccine	Administered every 6 to 10 years; begin at age 65 unless having lung disease, diabetes, or immune system compromise			Prevention of morbidity / mortality from complications of or as a direct result of infection from pneumococcal pneumonia	
	Tetanus vaccine /booster	Every ten years			Prevention of infection from clostridium tetani bacteria (lockjaw)	
	Influenza vaccine	Administered yearly, begin at age 65 unless having lung disease, diabetes, or immune system is compromised			Prevention of morbidity / mortality from complications of or as a direct result of infection from influenza virus	
	Colonoscopy	Everyone age ≥ 50 yrs. or earlier if family member with colorectal cancer prior to age 60 yrs. or have polyps or inflammatory bowel disease.			Prevention of colorectal cancer. Early detection reduces morbidity / mortality and optimizes outcomes.	

Mammogram	At age 40 or above; if positive family history, at discretion of gynecologist or PCP (usually sooner)	Prevention of breast cancer, early detection reduces morbidity/mortality and optimizes outcomes.
Pap smear	Begin when sexually active or no later than age 21 yrs. If after age 30, 3 consecutive negative Paps every 2 to 3 yrs.	Prevention of cervical cancer. Early detection reduces morbidity/mortality and optimizes outcomes.
DEXA scan / Bone Densitometry	All female patients over 65 and over; high risk males.	Prevention and treatment of osteoporosis[4]. Early detection reduces chance for fractures.
PSA level	Begin PSA[5] blood test at age 50 or sooner if symptoms present or at PCP's discretion.	Prevention of prostate cancer. Early detection reduces morbidity/mortality and optimizes outcomes. PSA less than 4.0 or at discretion of PCP.
Vision examination	Yearly if diabetic by ophthalmologist. If symptomatic, at discretion of PCP.	Optimize vision/quality of life; prevent accidents due to poor vision.
Dental examination	Daily flossing / regular brushing. If symptomatic at discretion of PCP.	Optimize dentition; improve quality of life.
Hearing examination	If symptomatic, see an ENT or audiologist	Optimize quality of life; prevent accidents resulting from poor hearing.

FOOT NOTES

1) PCP – Primary Care Physician.

2) Regarding NCEP guidelines, risk factors for cardiovascular disease include hypertension, diabetes, high cholesterol, smoking, sedentary lifestyle, family history, microalbuminuria.
NCEP guidelines for diabetics or those with a history of a heart attack or stroke are as follows:
HDL of > 40 if male   HDL>50 if female   LDL of < 70   Triglycerides of < 150

3) Diabetes testing can be done with:
a) random glucose level
b) glucose tolerance test
c) Hgb A1-C.

4) High risk for osteoporosis includes:
a) post-menopausal state without hormone replacement therapy
b) age over 60 years
c) low-activity lifestyle
d) low body weight
e) tobacco use
f) excessive alcohol intake
g) excessive caffeine intake
h) low calcium and vitamin D intake
i) medications
j) low testosterone levels in males.

5) PSA—Prostate Specific Antigen

CHAPTER NINE

LEGAL ISSUES IN MEDICINE

The medical field, like many other fields, is not void of legal issues. Many situations arise where having a reasonable understanding of the law will enable you to be prepared to respond in a crisis situation in the most appropriate manner and in the best interest of the involved party. There unfortunately can be no clearer example of the value of understanding the legal issues in medicine than the well-known case of Terry Schiavo. The importance of an advance directive can be no clearer than in this tragic case.

An advance directive is simply a document which, when becoming an official legal document, clearly states an individual's wishes regarding decisions to be made in his or her absence, or in situations where the individual is unable to decide for her or himself. This absence is usually the result of the individual's death or the result of the individual becoming incapable of making her own decisions. There are situations where an individual's ability to make decisions regarding his own affairs may become impaired. For example, an individual may lose consciousness due to trauma or a medical condition, and the need to have a life-saving aggressive measure may occur. At this point, if he is prepared with an advance directive giving specific instructions on how to make these important decisions, he not only guides the individual with the appointed decision-making capability (also known as the individual with durable power-of-attorney), but he also allows the decisions that have to be made to be made in accordance with his wishes.

A hypothetical situation which helps to illustrate this point is as in the following situation: A 40-year-old married man collapses at his home after reporting the acute onset of a severe headache. This man is rushed to the hospital and subsequent testing reveals a massive brain hemorrhage. He is then rushed to surgery where the brain hemorrhage is stabilized. After several days following the surgery, the man remains on life support in a comatose state. After being seen by a neurologist, it is felt that this man would not recover, and if indeed the man did recover, his quality of life would be very poor. At the present time, the man is being kept alive by artificial measures (the ventilator). Fortunately for both the man and his wife, the patient had an advance directive which stated that in the event that he became incapacitated and with little to no chance of a meaningful recovery or of a reasonable quality of life, he wished to not continue being maintained on artificial life support and to be allowed to expire with comfort measures only. At this point, the man's wife, although overcome with sorrow and despair, makes the decision to remove life support and to allow for comfort measures only in accordance with her spouse's wishes. The man expires shortly thereafter.

This previous example illustrates the numerous advantages made possible by having had a prepared advance directive. This made decision-making very clear for the person with durable power-of-attorney which was the spouse. It made clear the man's wishes in the event that he became incapacitated, as he unfortunately did. The fact that the decision to withdraw artificial life support was the decision of the victim helped to absolve feelings of guilt experienced by the man's spouse.

An advance directive can prove very useful in other situations as well. As in the case described above, for instance, imagine that family members of the man who suffered the brain hemorrhage arrive from out of town and demand that every measure be taken to keep him alive. Their demands, of course, are based on their own wishes as opposed to those of their dying relative. This dispute is clearly resolved as a result of two factors. Factor number one: A legal document, the advance directive, clearly states the person's (the man with the brain hemorrhage) wishes—in the event that he is incapacitated with a poor chance of recovery and/or that he is left with a poor quality of life—that comfort care measures without the use of artificial means of life support be implemented. Factor number two: The spouse, who has durable power-of-attorney in this case, has made the decision to honor the wishes outlined by her spouse.

Unfortunately, in the high-profile case of Terry Schiavo, an advance directive was not available in writing, and no one will ever know what her actual wishes were. It is unfortunate that most Americans in their thirties and forties do not have an advance directive in the event of a tragic, unexpected situation, as individuals do not expect to find themselves in such situations at this age. If you think about it, had the unfortunate Terry Schiavo had an advance directive, no one would even know who Terry Schiavo was. The case would have never escalated to the level that it did, and it would have saved Mrs. Schiavo's family enormous amounts of grief, financial resources, and time. For whatever it is worth, the anguish and suffering of the family of Terry Schiavo did indeed serve a meaningful purpose, if only to make more individuals aware of the importance of incorporating an advance directive as part of their preparedness for an unexpected tragic event.

An advance directive can be divided into two components: (1) a living will and (2) durable power-of-attorney. A living will, from a health-care standpoint, essentially is a legal document which states an individual's wishes regarding end-of-life situations. The purpose of having a legal document is to honor the wishes of the individual in a situation where he or she may be incapacitated. The living will serves as a guide for physicians in decision-making in patient management. Of particular importance and usefulness to the physician is a document known as a DNR which stands for "do not resuscitate." This particular document serves as a guide to the physician in situations where a patient is near death and the decision to continue life-saving measures has different possible approaches. The physician uses the information from the details outlined in the DNR order to guide him or her in choosing the management pathway which the patient would most likely have desired. With regard to a durable power-of-attorney, this is simply a document which appoints a specific person to act on behalf of the individual in the event that he or she becomes incapacitated. The individual with durable power-of-attorney is empowered with important decision-making authority on behalf of the incapacitated individual. These decisions are in reference to situations regarding, for the most part, end-of-life decisions. The individual appointed with durable power-of-attorney is chosen by the individual whom he or she represents. The person with durable power-of-attorney is usually, though not necessarily, a family member. Durable power-of-attorney is activated when the individual to whom it pertains becomes incapacitated (a determination that is made by a physician). As long as a person is capable of decision-making, no durable power-of-attorney is official or necessary.

The question now is how to obtain an advance directive. The answer is actually very simple. Advance directives can be obtained without the services of an attorney. You can simply download advance directive forms specific to your state off of the Internet. A very simple way to obtain advance directive forms is to do a search using Google (or any search engine for that matter), and look for the forms specific to the state in which you reside. These forms are essentially ready-made with a fill-in-the-blank format. In addition, you may add specifics to the document if additional wishes are desired. The important point is that you be clear about your wishes with regard to these end-of-life decisions. This can be best accomplished by clearly and accurately filling in the blanks and adding any details necessary to ascertain that your wishes be carried out as outlined. If you are uncertain as to whether the advance directive is actually legally binding, you should obtain counsel from an attorney just to be on the safe side.

One of the documents included in the advance directive is the DNR form. The DNR form, as previously mentioned, is a directive which outlines what measures are to be taken or not taken in the event that you become incapacitated, and decisions are to be made regarding medical management. The DNR comes into play when, say for instance, a patient will be requiring artificial life support as a result of a deterioration in health status in order to survive a crisis. It is during this time that immediate important decisions are to be made. With an intact advance directive, in this case the DNR status, the decision to proceed with very aggressive measures versus no aggressive measures can be made with clarity and without dispute. It should be pointed out before preceding any further that there are numerous possible ways in which a DNR order can be structured. In other words, the DNR order does not have to be either a "do everything possible to save a life" or a "no heroic efforts, comfort care only." There are different degrees of aggressive measures which can be specified in the DNR document, as well as different degrees of "no heroic measures, comfort care only." For example, an elderly female, who we will refer to as Miss X, lives in a nursing home where she was relocated after having suffered a stroke which left the right side of her body paralyzed, although she improved with physical therapy. Miss X is still alert and oriented to person, place, and time. Miss X has a DNR directive which specifies that in the event she should suffer a cardiac or pulmonary arrest, she would not want to be placed on life support (specifically on a ventilator/breathing machine), although it would be permissible to give drugs such as epinephrine or atropine in an effort to save her life. In reference to durable power-of-attorney, you must carefully select the individual to whom this role is awarded. When selecting your proxy (the individual empowered with durable power-of-attorney), you must realize that this individual will be making decisions which involve your own life and death. In other words, these are decisions of the utmost importance. Therefore, criteria should be established so as to achieve the best possible outcomes. It is suggested that the following criteria be considered when selecting an individual to which durable power-of-attorney is to be awarded:

1. An individual who is reliable and available. These qualities often go hand in hand. The concept is very simple. If the person you are considering is not reliable, it would be pointless to proceed any further. Very similarly, an individual who is unavailable is virtually worthless as a proxy, and awarding such an individual with durable power-of-attorney would be senseless.

2. An individual who has the strength to make a decision in a manner which honors you and your wishes. This quality is particularly important in the face of opposition which may come from both family and friends. Therefore, if this appointed proxy is easily swayed from acting according to directions, the outcome will not be in accordance with your wishes.

3. An individual (the proxy) who understands your outlook on life. In other words, someone who knows you well in order to act in the way which he or she feels that you would act in different situations. This will optimize the likelihood that your wishes will be carried out.

4. An individual who remains rational in difficult situations. This becomes very important as situations may become complicated, and are most likely to be quite stressful. In such situations, you would hope that your proxy would not succumb to pressure under but would rather remain level-headed. Such a stable proxy will, again, ensure that your wishes will be carried out.

Having discussed the important points involved in appointing a proxy, we will now consider what it means to actually be a proxy. As a proxy, there are obviously some helpful bits of information to consider when certain situations arise. For example, a 75-year-old female who has a history of multiple medical problems including diabetes, coronary artery disease, and high blood pressure presents to the emergency room with a deteriorating mental status. Subsequent workup in the emergency room reveals that this patient, who will be referred to as Mrs. Smith, has a urinary tract infection which has spread to the bloodstream causing her to become septic and near death. In order to save her life, she will require life support, at least initially. Mrs. Smith is a widow and has designated her daughter as her proxy. Mrs. Smith has an advance directive which states that in the event that she should become incapacitated and that her situation would leave a low likelihood of a reasonable quality of life if artificially kept alive, even if only temporarily, that she only be kept comfortable and that no heroic measures such as artificial life support be given. It should be mentioned that prior to this sudden illness, Mrs. Smith was living alone and independently. Now, imagine that you are the daughter who has durable power-of-attorney, and within ten minutes of arriving at the emergency room, you are approached by hospital personnel who want a decision on whether to give life support or not. What would be the important factors to take into consideration? The first thing you should do is take a deep breath and calm down as much as possible. Now, you need to consider Mrs. Smith's quality of life prior to the sudden deterioration in health. As was mentioned, Mrs. Smith was living alone and independently. Another thing to consider is if Mrs. Smith survives, will she have a reasonable quality of life? The answer to this question is most likely yes. Therefore, in this particular case, as a proxy, it would be reasonable to allow for artificial life support to be given, as it still is in compliance with the patient's wishes as clearly stated in her advance directive. In the event that Mrs. Smith has a poor hospitalization course, the decision to continue with artificial life support can be reevaluated at a later time.

The above scenario illustrates one of the many possible case scenarios and some helpful hints which may help you, if you are ever assigned as a proxy, to make some very critical decisions. In the case of Mrs. Smith, imagine for example that you, the proxy, felt pressured by the hospital personnel to discontinue life support when Mrs. Smith failed to improve enough after several days. You allow them to begin weaning her off life support, but then have second thoughts about it. What, if any, are your options? To begin with, you, as a proxy, should not make a decision that is so important based on feeling pressured. If those feelings exist, the option of reversing the decision and allowing for continuation of life support is a viable one. It is very important to know that advance directives can be changed at any given moment at the request of either the patient or the proxy (if the patient is incapacitated). Additionally, some degree of decision-making criteria should be given to your "gut feeling" about the situation. As different case scenarios arise, this feeling can be yet another tool to assist a proxy in making decisions.

Other aspects of decision-making in reference to advance directives are those of organ donation. It is ideal for this issue to be addressed in the advance directive, as it is a difficult decision to make under the stress of a crisis. Therefore, if these wishes are addressed and are made clear in advance, a huge burden is lifted from the proxy, particularly if the decision to donate organs was affirmative. Also, making a yes decision to organ donation minimizes any delays in the harvesting of organs in a situation where time is critical.

In the event that an advance directive has indicated comfort care, should the emergency situation arise, it is important to be aware of hospice services. Hospice is a service that is designed specifically for individuals who have been diagnosed with a terminal illness, are not expected to live more than six months, and have decided that no further heroic measures are to be taken. These heroic measures mean artificial life support and any further inpatient hospital care. It may be mentioned that if a patient lives more than the six months that were anticipated, hospice services can possibly be extended. Another item worth mentioning is that if a person has cancer, many hospice programs will not allow for chemotherapy, so if the patient wishes to continue with chemotherapy, oftentimes, hospice will not be an option.

In the preceding chapters, pertinent topics have been elaborated upon in an effort to provide the information necessary to enable you to optimize your health. The objectives of health are essentially two-fold with the first objective being to live a longer life and the second objective being to live a life of reasonable quality. Helpful criteria were outlined on how to select the primary care physician most suitable for you. Access to health care was discussed which described different types of insurance plans enabling you to choose the one most suitable for you. Helpful suggestions were provided which would result in a more productive office visit with your physician. The objectives of preventive medicine were clearly stated with detailed instruction on how to reach them. Health care issues regarding preventive medicine for three different age ranges were then discussed with accompanying charts making for a more organized approach to implement those preventive measures. Lastly, legal issues regarding end-of-life decisions such as those documented in living wills and the appointing of power of attorney were discussed so as to make for a more complete understanding of health care from beginning to end, ultimately providing an organized approach to optimizing your health.

ABOUT THE AUTHOR

Joseph A. Marotta, M.D. is a graduate of the University of Texas at Houston Medical School. He completed his residency training in Internal Medicine at Temple University Hospital in Philadelphia, Pennsylvania. He is board certified in Internal Medicine and has been in private practice in San Antonio, Texas for over ten years.

978-0-595-41091-0
0-595-41091-X

www.ingramcontent.com/pod-product-compliance
Lightning Source LLC
Chambersburg PA
CBHW030845180526
45163CB00004B/1448